Blueprint for Medical Care

The MIT Press
Cambridge, Massachusetts, and London, England

Blueprint for Medical Care

David D. Rutstein

Copyright © 1974 by
The Massachusetts Institute of Technology

All rights reserved. No part of this book may be reproduced in any form or by any means, electronic or mechanical, including photocopying, recording, or by any information storage and retrieval system, without permission in writing from the publisher.

This book was set in CRT Baskerville
printed on Mohawk Neotext Offset
and bound in G.S.B. S/535/151 "Navy"
by The Colonial Press Inc.
in the United States of America

ISBN 0-262-18065-0
Library of Congress catalog card number: 73-21474

Contents

Foreword by Jerome B. Wiesner   xi

Preface   xix

Introduction   1
The Blueprint   1
A Basic Assumption   2

1 The Institutional Structure   5
Background   5
Toward the Hospital of the Future   7

2 A Regional System   15
Lines of Communication and Transportation within a Regional System   20
The People Served (Well and Sick)   20
Physicians and Allied Health Personnel   22
Transportation of Laboratory Specimens   24

Contents   vi

3 Information Processing   27
Individual Patient Care   27
Clinical Research   31
Patient Scheduling   32
Administrative Operation   33
Professional Education   34
Allied Medical Professions   35
Electronic Signals   36
A Practical Example: Consultation at a Distance   37
Methods of Communication for Consultation within a Regional System   44
The Region: The Operating Unit for Medical Care   46

4 The Medical Manpower Muddle   52
The Solution of the Manpower Muddle   58

5 Emergency Medical Care: The First Step   62
The Military Experience in Emergency Care   66
A Regional Emergency Program   67
The Emergency Communications Network   69
The Transportation System   71

6 Ambulatory Medical Care: The Unfilled Gap   80
Private Care   82
   The Private Individual Physician   82
   Private Physicians in a Group Practice Unit   84
Institutional Ambulatory Care   86
   Ambulatory Care Clinics   86
Medical Care Programs for Disadvantaged Populations   87

Contents vii

Double Standard of Medical Care 89
Scarcity of General Physicians 90

7 **The Ambulatory Program of the Future** 92
Where Shall the Patient Be Treated? 93
The Composite Plan 97
Essential Elements of an Ambulatory Program 98
The Treatment Center 99

8 **The General Physician: The "Captain of the Team"** 103
The Trend from General Physician to Specialist 112
The Rebirth of the General Physician 114
The Different Roles of General Physician and Specialist 116

9 **The Reception Center** 119
Patient Referral System in Ambulatory Care 120
Allied Health Services 128
Preventive Services 129
School Health Services 130
First Aid and Minor Care 130
Home Visiting Services 131

10 **Communication and Transportation Systems** 133

11 **Medical Education for the Future** 139
The Changing Pattern of Medical Education 139
A Multichannel Curriculum: The Only Solution 142

Criteria for the Medical Curriculum   143
A. The Pathways   144
B. Transfer among Pathways   146
C. A Continuous Curriculum   147
D. Variation in Basic Courses   149
E. A Balanced Education   150
F. The Total Length of the Curriculum   151
G. Qualifications for Admission to Medical Education   152
H. Awarding of Degrees   158

The Curriculum for the General Physician   159

12 The Quality of Medical Care   161

Existing Standards, Procedures, and Indices of Health and Medical Care   163
Qualifications of Medical Personnel   163
Institutional Medical Care   165
Indices of Health in the General Population   169

13 Quality Control Systems   174

The Guidance System   175
Implementation of the Guidance System   185
Unnecessary Disease   185
Unnecessary Disability   187
Unnecessary Untimely Death   187
Medical Resources and Flow Patterns of Disease, Disability, and Death   189

Feasibility of a Guidance System   189
The Early Warning System   191

14 Converting the Numbers into Better Health   199

The Federal Health Board   200
Not an Administrative Agency   204
Structure and Membership   205

Regional Health Boards 207
Duties of the
Federal Health Board 208
1. Guide the Conversion into the National Health Program 209
2. Assay National and Regional Health, and Pinpoint Measures for Improvement 213
3. Establish New Indices of Health 214
4. Document Scientific, Professional, and Technical Evaluations of Medicine, Medical Care, and Health 216
5. Recommend Priorities in Expenditure of the National Health Budget to Attain Highest Possible Levels of Health 218
6. Identify National Health Emergencies and Local Health Emergency Areas 220
7. Develop a National Health Code 220
8. Establish Liaison with the Congressional Office of Health Care 222

15 **The Public Interest** 225

At the National Level 226
At the Local Level 228
The Education Program 229
Education of the Staff 231
The Health Alerting System 232

16 **Payment to the Physician** 236

Proposed Method of Payment 238

17 **Administration** 242

A Historical Note 242
The Recommended Model 246
The Implementation 248
Local Health Administration 250

18 Financing Medical Care   254
The Insurance Principle   254
Federal Insurance   255
Proposed Method of Financing   258

19 The Crucial Question   262
Appendix   265

Index   277

List of Figures

Figure 1. The hospital of the future   6
Figure 2. The regional system   16
Figure 3. Ambulatory care   49
Figure 4. Administrative structure for a national health program   249

Foreword

The shortcomings in our medical care system become dramatically evident to the average citizen when illness strikes close to home. He is stymied by unbelievable disorganization with lack of clear-cut entry points to care, particularly at night, on weekends, and on holidays. He is overwhelmed by the skyrocketing costs of illness, especially when admission to a hospital becomes necessary. He is appalled by the obstructions to care due to such factors as his geographic location, the per capita income and urbanization of his neighborhood, and his accessibility to a medical center.

The resulting crisis has precipitated a number of private health care plans, and a spectrum of legislative proposals for the development of a national health program. All promise better health for Americans. Because of the great difficulty in identifying critical limiting factors and in proposing politically acceptable remedies, the bills that have been introduced in the Congress are

Foreword

primarily concerned with the insurance and administrative aspects of a national health program. The essential details of implementation and evaluation tend to be hidden under general terms such as health maintenance organizations, medical foundations, and peer review. It is not clear as to how the establishment of any or all of these agencies will actually improve the health of the average American. Indeed, a major reason for the delay in the enactment of national health legislation is the lack of a specific professional and technical plan of medical care delivery to serve as a basis for agreement.

I believe that Doctor Rutstein's plan could fill this gap. His blueprint proposes a plan for integrating the individual units of a national health program into a complete system. Most important, it makes provision for critical review, testing, and evaluation so that modification and improvement may be effected without delay as experience and research results are accumulated. The plan incorporates a quality control system that can measure the effect of the operation of the separate units of the program on the health of the population. The blueprint is not and cannot be a final plan for a national health program for the United States. But it can serve as a good beginning. It provides a description of the course of program evolution and operation and an estimate of its potential impact upon individual and national health. Especially significant is the fact that it can be the focus for national discussion among all concerned and serve as a basis for legislative agreement.

In terms of practical implementation, Doctor Rutstein on the final page of the blueprint has raised "The

Crucial Question": "How can our complex society suppress its primitive fear of change and use our treasure of existing knowledge, our army of educated and trained personnel, our superb institutional structures, our rapidly expanding technology, and our storehouse of social and financial resources, and rally the providers and consumers of medical care on the basis of enlightened self-interest to diminish suffering, postpone untimely death, and improve our individual and national health?" The practical answer to that question will depend upon political leadership that will achieve general agreement on the preliminary objectives and determine the first stages of the implementation of a national health program.

It is easy to recognize the difficulty of motivating the various groups who must collaborate to create a national health system. There is little to be learned from the processes by which the various existing national care systems such as those in the United Kingdom or the Soviet Union came into existence because both the social settings and the economic situations in which they emerged were so different from ours. Americans desire to preserve the advantages of diversity and choice for the recipients of care and a challenging spectrum of opportunities for those who choose to become professionals in the health care field. This requires reconciling institutional integrity and conformity with the dictates of local and regional needs of the health care system. For example, the superspecialist in the medical school hospital, without being hampered in his essential research and teaching, will provide his uncommon but often life-saving services to everyone needing them in the region with which his hospital is affiliated.

Doctor Rutstein proposes to begin with regional consolidation and improvement of the emergency care components of the health care system on the grounds that they are so thoroughly inadequate and chaotic that it should be relatively easy to mobilize support for this step. It should be possible to make a dramatic demonstration of the value of a coherent system in this aspect of medical care, for the gap between what is feasible and what exists is tremendous. Moreover, the lives of many hundreds of accident victims could undoubtedly be saved each year by making effective emergency care generally available. It is good that efforts toward this end are already under way throughout the country. But it is not obvious to me that the people of the United States should or will wait for a demonstration of an efficient emergency care system for the creation of a more effective general health maintenance and care program.

The quality control system in the blueprint was developed with the assistance and advice of the National Center for Health Statistics and the Center for Disease Control, and it should certainly be tested in the field. If those tests were successful, it would be desirable to institute that system as soon as possible so that the current state of health of the country would guide the evolution of the total national health program.

Throughout the blueprint, there are many other practical suggestions for immediate study or for implementation that do not require the organization of a national health program for their performance. These include an integrated health record for everyone, the definition of the roles of the physician and allied health personnel so that manpower estimates can be made with some confidence, the fitting together of a curriculum for the education of the general physician, and the development of the required instrumentation and systems organization for communication and transportation. There is no reason why areas such as these should not be explored immediately.

On the other side, I would be reluctant to legislate a comprehensive national medical system into existence in one fell swoop, for I doubt that we have either the manpower or the knowledge to do so. The nation's experience with housing programs and other large-scale social innovations should make us just a bit cautious. In addition to the national emergency care system, the quality control system, and the exploration of feasible subunits of a program, I would opt for a number of experiments chosen to provide experience in total medical care, as outlined in this blueprint, under all of the kinds of conditions in which such care has to be provided in the United States. Furthermore, the implementation of any plan should be based upon the availability of skilled manpower and facilities and should not be allowed to outrun the growth in these limiting factors. Otherwise the results are likely to be counterproductive.

The only reason for being at all hopeful about "voluntary" participation in a national health system that involves a high degree of coordination and self-discipline is the severe and growing financial problems of almost all institutional units of the health care system, hospitals, medical schools, and ambulatory and emergency services. Rational behavior may be more acceptable than bankruptcy. Moreover, it will take a high order of political leadership to ensure that the opportunities provided by the growing financial crisis are not undercut by a series of haphazardly developed independent federal health care programs that will provide little if any incentive toward an efficient national system. In this connection, some of the administrative elements of the blueprint—the Federal Health Board, the Congressional Office of Health Care, and the reorganization and expansion of the professional corps of the Department of Health, Education, and Welfare—deserve careful study at the highest level of government by competent commissions appointed for this purpose. Many of the proposed duties and responsibilities of these agencies will be essential in meeting acute crises and in supervising the professional, scientific, and technical elements, and in taking into account the public interest in the development of a national health program. Furthermore, implementing legislation will be needed to create and define the administrative elements essential to planning and operation of a national program. All of these efforts must be accompanied by an educational program for the public, the purveyors of medical care, and the governmental representatives of the people. Educated leadership and an informed public are a sine qua non for the planning and operation of a complete and efficient national system of medical care.

One final word might also be said about the blueprint

approach to social problems. It will be of interest to see whether this formulation of a national health program will lead to a successful outcome. One might also wonder whether the blueprint approach is not applicable to other pressing professional and technical social problems, such as mass urban transportation, that must be solved if our civilization is to survive and prosper.

Jerome B. Wiesner
President
Massachusetts Institute of Technology

Cambridge, Massachusetts
August 1, 1973

Preface

This blueprint outlines a preventive and therapeutic medical care program to bring better health to the people of the United States. It is based on a series of lectures and related conferences in 1970–1971, when I was Visiting Institute Lecturer at the Massachusetts Institute of Technology. *Blueprint for Medical Care*, written for the layman, presents a single coherent plan interrelating the essential points of a total medical care program. The modular units of the program are separately defined so that they are amenable to constructive criticisms and suggestions by representatives of the many relevant disciplines concerned with medical care delivery. Moreover, the individual subunits can be studied by mathematical modeling and simulation and then redesigned for controlled testing and evaluation under actual field conditions. At a time when the establishment of a national health program seems imminent, the blueprint can serve as a guide to the design, operation, and evaluation of a total system of care to be constantly improved and expanded as experience and research results are accumulated. And we must begin now.

A proposal of a complete blueprint for medical care may be dismissed as being idealistic and impractical. But the actual situation is exactly the opposite. The costs of medical care are completely out of hand. Indeed, the total cost of medical care in the United States is increasing constantly and has already reached the staggering sum of over eighty billion dollars per year, equivalent to about 8.3 percent of gross national product. And, yet, in spite of the exponential trend, there is the constant complaint of inadequate funds for essential services, and many of our hospitals, both municipal and voluntary, are on the verge of bankruptcy. More important, the health status of the United States leaves very much to be desired. It is clear that the rising cost of medical care will, in itself, dictate major changes in the way that medicine will be practiced in the future. We must take advantage of this rare opportunity for optimal planning, which may be defined as efficient cooperation with the inevitable, to bring better health to the people of our country.

As we start to improve care, a single glance tells us that halfway measures will no longer suffice. Our patchwork quilt of medical care is beyond repair. Without any overall planning, we have added, higgledy-piggledy, to a crazy quilt of multiple systems, one patch after another—physicians' assistants, health maintenance organizations, emergency care, peer review, the Professional Standards Review Organization, and that patch with the hole in it—Medicaid. Patches lie upon patches, as in the case of physicians' assistants' services and nursing care, while the cold wind of unnecessary illness and death continues to blow through the unrepaired gaps and rents in our incomplete medical care system.

The lack of a single system of medical care has been an almost insurmountable obstacle to the improvement of the quality and efficiency of care for all Americans. The many different kinds of purveyors of care and insurance carriers have created endless confusion and an enormous waste in administrative cost. The purveyors include private practitioners, group practice units, and the outpatient departments and emergency care services of community, voluntary, municipal, proprietary, and university hospitals. The myriad of insurance carriers comprises Blue Cross-Blue Shield and private insurance companies, Medicare, Medicaid, and an almost infinite variety of federal, state, and local welfare and ghetto programs. It is inconceivable that high-quality efficient care for all can be provided without welding all of them and all other existing resources into a single system. And yet there is a continued demand for "pluralism" in the development of a national health program. Imagine how silly it would be to demand pluralism in urban telephone communication. To be sure, there must be an interim period when advantage is taken of all useful resources of existing agencies by gradually integrating them into a functional whole. It will be a great challenge to preserve their individual special contributions as they are merged into a total program. Thus, for example, the opportunities for leadership of our great voluntary hospitals such as the Massachusetts General Hospital in the improvement of inpatient care, and of ambulatory care by outstanding prepayment group practice units such as the Kaiser-Permanente Medical Care Program must be preserved at all costs. Moreover, as in countries with national health programs, such as the United Kingdom and Sweden, the private practice of medicine will continue to be available for those who wish to obtain their medical care in that fashion.

We do need a plan for a single prepaid national health program for everybody. That program should provide, through a personal physician relationship, the highest possible quality of preventive and therapeutic medical care by optimal application of our scientific knowledge, professional competence and skills, institutional facilities, and technology within the limitations of our economic, personnel, and social resources. This blueprint outlines such a plan and the details of its implementation. Moreover, it incorporates a system of quality control to monitor the health of the population served and to evaluate changes produced by the individual elements of the program. This blueprint does not presume to supply all of the details of a total national health and medical care program, but it does provide the basis upon which such a program may be planned, implemented, and evaluated in order to bring better health to all Americans.

Beginning with the pioneers, the late Dr. Joseph W. Mountin of the United States Public Health Service and the late Dr. John B. Grant of the Rockefeller Foundation, I am deeply indebted to many colleagues and friends within and without the medical profession who have over the years contributed ideas, facts, and critical discussions that have helped to clarify my thinking in the many disciplines relevant to medicine and to medical care delivery. They will understand that I can acknowledge only the assistance of those who have been of immediate help in the writing of this book. I particularly appreciate the thoughtful and constructive criticisms and suggestions following careful reading of this manuscript by Dr. George Baehr, Distinguished Service Professor, Mt. Sinai School of Medicine; Dr. Leona Baumgartner, Visiting Professor of Social Medicine, Harvard Medical School; Dr. Harvey Brooks, Dean, Division of Engineering and Applied Physics, Harvard University; Kingsbury Browne, Partner, Hill and Barlow; Dr. W. Palmer Dearing, former Executive Director, Group Health Association of America; Sir Richard Doll, Regius Professor of Medicine, University of Oxford; Murray Eden, Professor of Electrical Engineering, Massachusetts Institute of Technology; Dr. Charles C. Edwards, Assistant Secretary for Health, Department of Health, Education, and Welfare; Jack Feldman, Professor of Biostatistics, Harvard School of Public Health; Dr. Manfred L. Karnovsky, Harold T. White Professor of Biological Chemistry, Harvard Medical School; Dr. Alexander Leaf, Jackson Professor of Clinical Medicine, Harvard Medical School; Dr. Nathalie P. Masse, Director of Education, International Children's Center, Paris; George J. Nielson, Charles Stark Draper Laboratory; George St. John Perrott, formerly Chief, Division of Public Health Methods, Office of the Surgeon General; Lord Robert Platt, Professor of Medicine Emeritus, University of Manchester; Professor Bror Rexed, Director-General of

Preface   xxiv

the National Board of Health and Welfare, Sweden; Dr. David J. Sencer, Director, and Dr. Michael Lane, Assistant to Director, Center for Disease Control, Department of Health, Education, and Welfare; Dr. Charles A. Sanders, General Director, Massachusetts General Hospital; Eugene B. Skolnikoff, Professor and Chairman, Department of Political Science, Massachusetts Institute of Technology; and Theodore Woolsey, Director, National Center for Health Statistics, Department of Health, Education, and Welfare. Their contributions, many of which are incorporated into this book, are deeply appreciated with the understanding that I am solely responsible for the facts, their interpretation, and for any errors in the published text.

Special acknowledgment is made to Rita J. Nickerson, Research Associate in Preventive and Social Medicine, for keeping a watchful eye on the statistical interpretations in the text and for verifying the references; and to Emily P. Flint, former managing editor of *The Atlantic Monthly* for her meticulous and constructive editorial assistance. I also wish to thank Esta J. Lupo and Ernestine M. Dinis for typing the numerous drafts.

I am grateful to the Massachusetts Institute of Technology for the privilege of serving as Visiting Institute Lecturer in 1970–1971, when I explored with faculty and students many of the ideas that are put together here, and to The Commonwealth Fund for a grant for editorial expenses.

David D. Rutstein, M.D.
July 11, 1973

Blueprint for Medical Care

Introduction

The Blueprint

This blueprint of the structure and function of a national medical care[1] program will:

• define the institutional structure of the hospital of the future and its function in a regional system of health care;

• propose a design of areawide emergency medical care systems to serve as the first step in the evolution of a complete medical care program;

• indicate how our major gap in medical care, ambulatory services, may be repaired by a new system—coordinated with acute and chronic inpatient hospital facilities within a regional structure and with a more efficient use of medical manpower and modern technology so as to assure earlier, continuous, and complete patient care;

• devise a medical education program to graduate both

1. In this blueprint, the term medical care includes dental care.

the general physicians needed for preventive, primary, personal, and continuing care of the patient and the specialists required to meet the increasingly complex demands of medical care, research, and education;
• create a quality and efficiency control system using direct measures of the quality of medical care, cost effectiveness data on the efficiency of care, and estimates of the optimal potential for care which are based on the store of medical scientific knowledge and technology, the availability of professional competence and skills, and the sum of economic, institutional, and social resources to guide the expenditure of funds for preventive and therapeutic services toward maximal improvement of national health;
• outline the legislative requirements and the consumer participation and education that could take advantage of the planned and systematic use of our national resources in order to attain our goal of optimal health for all of our citizens;
• suggest a method of payment to physicians that recognizes their special contributions to society and yet permits precise estimates of total annual costs for physician services that must be covered in a complete medical care insurance program;
• define an administrative structure and method of financing that would bring all of the elements together into a unified national health program.

A Basic Assumption
The proposal of a defined medical care system arouses fears of increasing depersonalization of medical care.

A Basic Assumption

Visions are conjured up of a patient being diagnosed by a computer and treated by a robot. The fears are not groundless. Some health plans completely neglect the personal aspects of health care. But let us not be misled. In our present catch-as-catch-can lack of system, many Americans do not now have a personal physician and their proportion grows progressively larger as time goes on. The trend must be reversed.

The heart of the proposed medical care system is a personal physician relationship to offer guidance, reassurance, and support to the patient. Any system that destroys that relationship cannot provide complete medical care. The system by itself must not take over. Good medical care will not be provided by the automatic collection of reams of information of questionable reliability and of varying degrees of relevance, or by the random ordering of batteries of laboratory tests, or by fixed rigid patterns of treatment. The physician, or his surrogate in a remote rural area, must take charge and decide which of the resources of the system will be needed for his patient. At times, it will be essential for the physician to protect his patient against the system by preventing meddlesome interference implicit in the performance of a risky unnecessary laboratory test or the administration of inappropriate therapy, such as the treatment of a common cold with an antibiotic.

As this blueprint unfolds, it will become clear that it is proposed to increase the number of general physicians, to assign to them the role of "captain of the team," and to allocate to them the responsibility for primary, personal, and continuous care for each individual patient. Moreover, each person must have complete freedom of choice of physician among all those available in his area. Indeed, if this blueprint were implemented most patients might well look forward in the future to having a "doctor of their own" and of their own choice practicing within an efficient medical care system.

The Institutional Structure 1

Background

During the first half of the twentieth century, the hospital changed from a custodial institution to a complex workshop. By the turn of the next century, it will incorporate personnel, technology, and services for preventive and curative medicine; and will become the center of community health. The projected regional institutional structure in our blueprint will be built around our present hospitals. But first, community hospitals must be redesigned into the community health centers of the future, and their activities must be coordinated with those of the adjacent medical school hospital into a functioning regional system.

Our hospitals have been proud, self-centered institutions which have evolved haphazardly, often with little regard to community needs. In a word, our hospitals act in isolation and try to be completely self-sufficient instead of collaborating in the total health service of the commu-

The Institutional Structure

Figure 1. The hospital of the future.

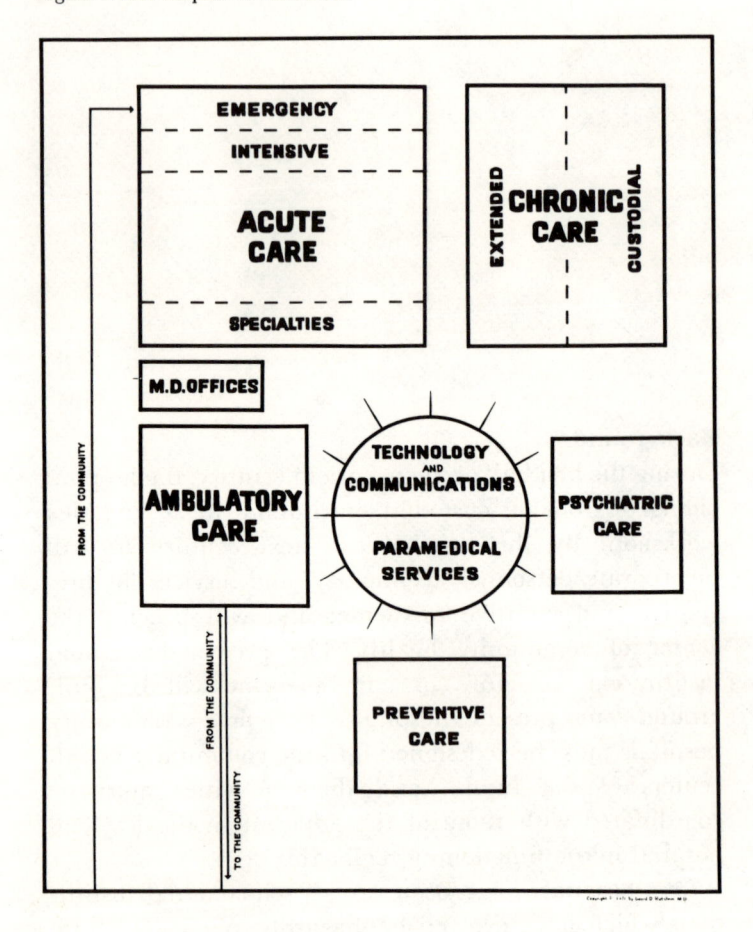

nity. Their growth and excellence have depended upon the breadth of vision of their trustees, the drive of their medical staff, and the generosity of their private and governmental donors. Most university and community hospitals have neglected the ambulatory care of patients as they have concentrated on the care of the acutely ill patient in the horizontal position in bed. Indeed, American hospitals provide for severely ill patients inpatient services as good as or better than any in the world. Moreover, in their zeal, individual hospitals continue to increase their superspecialist services for inpatients, as they compete with others in the same community to be the first to add a cobalt bomb or an open-heart surgical or a coronary care unit. Costly technological facilities are frequently purchased for the convenience of the staff even though the community may already have a surfeit of such resources. Preference tends to be given to the more newsworthy procedures such as heart transplants while ambulatory care continues to be chaotic, whole population groups in ghetto areas are neglected, and more important but less dramatic preventive services are overlooked. In a word, the modern hospital in its present form is not designed to provide complete and continuous medical care to all of its patients.

Toward the Hospital of the Future

The institutional structure of American medicine will need to be changed. The hospital of the future (figure 1) should be community-centered and not self-centered and should carry out its defined share of the total medical program. All commonly required medical care personnel and facilities should be located within the community hospital and should include all general physicians, frequently used specialists, allied medical personnel, and modern technology in the form of a true group practice unit. They should all be effectively interrelated at the hospital site to provide up-to-date, high-quality, continuous care. Concentrating ambulatory services at the community hospital will eliminate the existing chaos and fragmentation and their diffusion throughout the community in doctors' offices, group practice units, isolated clinics, hospital outpatient departments, and emergency wards. Moreover, ambulatory care will be available in the community hospital when really needed at all hours of the day and night, on weekends and holidays, so that a patient would no longer be forced to turn to a chiropractor, the local druggist, or a next-door neighbor for care that should be provided by a physician. The concentration of resources at the hospital will require that effective communication and transportation systems in both rural and urban areas be established connecting the patient's home with district reception centers and community hospitals so that each resident of the community, when he really needs his personal physician, will have immediate access to him or to his stand-in in the group practice unit in the community hospital. In this new institutional structure, the physician will, in turn, have access to all the resources necessary to meet his patients' preventive and therapeutic medical needs.

As in the past, the community hospital will provide inpatient care for the acutely ill. But its responsibility will not end there. As patients recover from acute illness, they will be transferred when required for convalescent care to adjacent completely adequate, but less expensive, extended care facilities. Moreover, chronically ill patients, sick enough to require continuing institutional care will no longer be shunted out of the hospital to be forgotten in those nonmedical institutions called nursing homes. Instead, they will be transferred within the hospital to appropriate and accessible custodial care facilities. There would then be no need for the conscientious physician to waste valuable professional time driving hither and yon to care for his chronically ill patients. With access to all of the commonly required resources within the community hospital, the physician would provide better and more effective care to all of his patients.

One major class of chronic illness deserves special mention. Patients with psychiatric disease have been banished to remote, enormous, impersonal custodial institutions, most of which are short of resident staffs, general physicians, specialists, and nurses, as well as psychiatrists. In the community hospital of the future, psychiatry will be brought into the mainstream of medicine. Both inpatient and ambulatory services are needed to cover the entire range of mental disease. Depending upon the needs of the individual patient, a series of graded services would be developed extending all the way from intermittent ambulatory care for patients living in their own homes to part- or full-time hospital care. In psychiatric units within the community hospital of the future, the patient will become more readily accessible to his physician, allied medical personnel, technological resources, his psychiatrist, and his family. Indeed, the patient, during the entire course of his therapy, will be seen through the eyes of a physician as well as those of a psychiatrist, with a better balance of medical and psychiatric care than is now available in isolated custodial institutions. Merely bringing the psychiatric patient back into society may help to assuage his hopelessness so that he may cooperate more effectively with those responsible for his care.

The platitude that prevention is better than treatment is constantly repeated but generally ignored. Most of our community hospitals, except for their obstetric and pediatric services, have abdicated their preventive responsibility and have relinquished it to the health office in city hall. It is time that prevention be made an integral part of medical care. Accumulating medical knowledge has blurred and is now obliterating the line between preventive and curative medicine. Modern preventive medicine must be transferred from city hall into the hospital and the position of health officer merged with that of hospital administrator. These changes will require the education of a new kind of health administrator.

The preventive point of view must also be introduced into the day-by-day practice of medical care. Well-baby care, immunization, and the epidemiologic control of the spread of infectious disease both within the hospital and in the surrounding community must be extended to the prevention of noninfectious disease, particularly those man-made diseases resulting from hazardous occupations, pollution, radiation, accidents, drug reactions, exposure to artificial environments (sealed air-conditioned buildings and caissons at the bottom of a river) and the iatrogenic diseases, that is, illnesses created by doctors. Other kinds of preventive services within the hospital would include the screening for previously unrecognized diseases that are better treated early than late,[1] for example, cancer of the rectum or high blood pressure, the anticipation and forestalling of serious complications of acute and chronic illness, and the rehabilitation of the handicapped. The wise leavening of preventive judgment must become a permanent part of the management of all patients at all stages of disease.

Figure 1 identifies individual services and their interrelationships in the hospital of the future. It must be clear that it does not specify the actual building arrangements on the hospital grounds. Thus, while the doctors' offices, the emergency care facilities, the ambulatory care unit, and preventive services are diagrammed as separate units, it is likely that for purposes of efficiency they might well be all housed together in a group practice unit in the same building with easy access to the technological resources and allied medical personnel of the inpatient services. The details of this blueprint will, of course, have to be adapted by each community to consumer and political pressures and to such local considerations as the population served, economic resources, existing hospital structures, and geographic factors, deviating as little as possible, however, from the pursuit of the overall objective of high-quality, efficient medical care as measured

1. D. D. Rutstein, "Screening Tests in Mass Surveys and Their Use in Heart Disease Case Finding," *Circulation* 4 (November 1951): pp. 659–665.

by a minimal level of unnecessary disease, disability, and untimely death.

Hospital reorganization uniting isolated medical care units dispersed throughout the community into a single site may require the purchase of adjacent land. Some of the expansion will be offset by replacing the relatively large space occupied by unnecessary hospital beds by less space-demanding ambulatory care services. For the community as a whole, some of the increased land costs will be compensated for by the closing of isolated institutions such as nursing homes. In the long run, the increased capital investment will be more than justified by the savings in professional time and the improvement in the efficiency, continuity, and decency of individual patient care.

The self-centered community hospital still tries by itself to provide all of the services needed by every patient. But as time goes on, that role becomes less and less feasible. There are many examples. It has long been understood that the laboratories of every hospital cannot perform all required tests. Complicated, unusual, and dangerous laboratory tests have been farmed out to laboratories in other hospitals and in state health departments, to mail-order commercial laboratories, or to unique laboratories such as that of the Center for Disease Control, Department of Health, Education, and Welfare in Atlanta, Georgia. In epidemic emergencies, hospital resources have been centralized for their most effective use. Thus, in the polio epidemic in metropolitan Boston in 1955, three hospitals were selected to treat all of the patients under the supervision of a few eminent specialists. The patients received superb care. In recent years, because of an oversupply of maternity and pediatric beds and a falling birth rate, some hospitals have discontinued their obstetrical or pediatric services, and some have discontinued both. In the use of complicated, expensive, newly developed life-saving equipment such as the artificial kidney, there has been some tendency to concentrate the service in a few hospitals in each community. In contrast, in many hospitals, particularly in our larger cities, there has been an almost endless proliferation of such highly specialized services as the radiation treatment of cancer, open-heart surgery, and intensive care and coronary care units.

The tendency to provide complete medical care in every hospital has been harmful as well as expensive because in most community hospitals, uncommon superspecialist procedures are not performed often enough to maintain, let alone upgrade, the skills of the superspecialists. For example, a recent analysis of surgery of congenital heart disease in hospitals in New England has demonstrated that the death rates for each type of operation are as much as two and one-half times as high in some hospitals, as in others.[2] It is not uncommon to see a superspecialist in a suburban hospital using special equipment purchased at great expense by the local community and attempting to carry out an unusual procedure which can be more safely and effectively performed in the nearby urban medical center. Local pride and individual initiative are laudable virtues, but

2. D. C. Fyler, "The New England Regional Infant Cardiac Program," personal communication (1973).

they must not cost the life or health of a patient. A superspecialist may provide irreplaceable life-saving care but relatively few patients will need his help. He must serve a large population if his knowledge is to continue to grow and if he is to keep his skills at peak efficiency. As a general principle, since no community hospital can provide every service, it becomes clear that hospitals must share their resources with one another if the patient is to get what he needs when he needs it.

A Regional System

2

We are thus faced with a dilemma. Not every hospital can provide but every patient should have whatever is required to bring to him in time of need the maximum benefits of modern medicine. There is only one solution. All hospitals in each medical services area must have their services so interrelated that the entire regional system should function as a single institution with appropriate division of labor among the constituent hospitals (figure 2). Each community hospital will be the focus of primary care where the patient's physician will be located and commonly used specialized services will be performed. In the central hospital, essential and expensive but uncommonly used technological resources and personnel will be concentrated in support of superspecialists' services, and wasteful, unnecessary duplication could be ended.

It is fortunate that most of the approximately one hundred medical schools and their teaching hospitals are

A Regional System

Figure 2. The regional system.

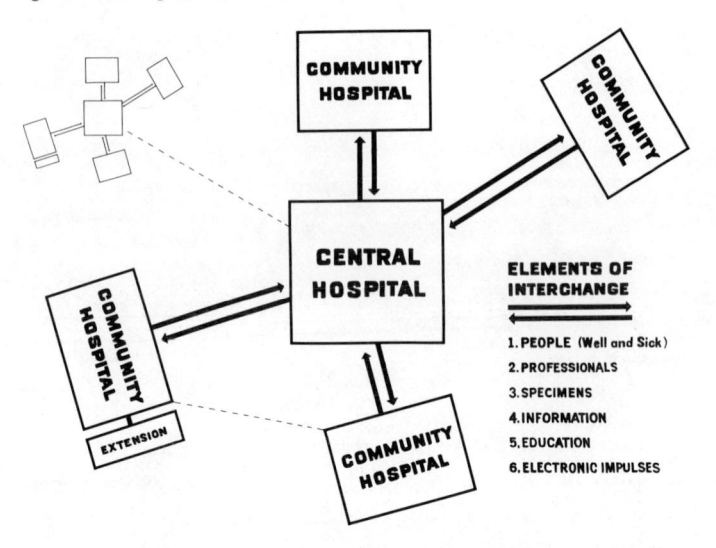

ELEMENTS OF INTERCHANGE

1. PEOPLE (Well and Sick)
2. PROFESSIONALS
3. SPECIMENS
4. INFORMATION
5. EDUCATION
6. ELECTRONIC IMPULSES

so distributed around the country that they could serve as the central hospitals in most of the proposed individual medical care regions of one to three million population. The establishment of new medical schools as authorized by Act of Congress,[1] to be affiliated with existing veterans hospitals, modified in accordance with the recommendations of the Deans Committees to the Veterans Administration after World War II,[2] could serve as central hospitals for the few remaining regions where medical

[1] "Veterans Administration Medical School Assistance and Health Manpower Training Act of 1972," Public Law 541, 92nd Congress.
[2] "Plans for Cooperation Between Teaching Institutions and Veterans' Hospitals," *Journal of the American Medical Association* 129 (December 15, 1945): pp. 1100–1102.

A Regional System

schools do not now exist (the State of Maine and the eastern slopes of the Rocky Mountains). In mapping regional systems, it would be desirable, insofar as possible, to make them congruent with established marketing and service areas so that the flow of individuals and information among the hospitals would be facilitated by existing communication and transportation systems.

The design of the central and community hospitals must be adapted to their respective roles. The initial decisions as to allocation of functions to each of them will have to be evaluated critically and modified as experience is accumulated and studies are performed. The individual elements (figure 1) in central and community hospitals will be the same, but the composition of each of the elements will vary depending on the hospital's role in the regional system. Thus, the community hospital will be concerned with giving the patient all usual medical care including initial diagnostic workups, ambulatory and inpatient care of acute episodes of illness, and the follow-up and management of chronic disease. Highly sophisticated and technical superspecialists' services will be provided in the central hospital where day-by-day care will be limited to patients whose illness demands supervision by superspecialists. Dialysis by an artificial kidney of acutely ill patients leading to kidney transplantation is an example. Functions that are intermediate between superspecialists and general services will have to be provisionally assigned pending the results of research studies and accumulated experience in the use of regional medical care systems.

A special word needs to be said about the functions of

A Regional System

a small isolated hospital in a very rural area—a cottage hospital—that will be set up as an extension or an affiliate of a distant community hospital (figure 2). The experience in northern Sweden above the Arctic Circle is instructive. Swedish cottage hospitals are not permitted to operate as individual institutions. Instead, their medical care is integrated with that of a parent community hospital even though it may be many miles away. Clear-cut policies have been established that limit the services provided within the cottage hospital to those that can be safely and effectively performed with the use of its resources. Defined minor illnesses are cared for locally in the cottage hospital. Patients with certain severe illnesses are automatically admitted as inpatients not to the local cottage hospital but to the distant community hospital. Patients with moderate illness are evaluated in the cottage hospital and decisions made as to the best location for treatment. The range of laboratory services in cottage hospitals has been specifically planned and defined and related to the number and kinds of available physicians and allied medical personnel so that the laboratory resources, by themselves, almost automatically determine the location of care for patients with illnesses of intermediate severity. Thus, illnesses whose treatment can be guided by the use of laboratory resources limited to simple procedures such as the counting and examination of blood cells and the analysis of the urine, and such routine biochemical measurements as a blood sugar determination are cared for within the cottage hospital. Patients are transferred to the community hospital when they have complicated illnesses which demand continuous precise laboratory monitoring for immediate patient management, or which require more sophisticated measurements such as the acid base balance of the blood, or complicated x-ray examinations, or which need highly specialized technicians to test, for example, the sensitivity to antibiotics of germs causing severe infections.

The efficient integration of the medical care programs of the community and cottage hospitals will demand highly efficient communication and transportation systems to assure early and effective treatment of all patients. In Sweden, patients are transferred by ambulances appropriately equipped and manned by drivers trained to perform such services as resuscitation, first aid, intravenous therapy, the application of splints, and the use of defibrillators and drugs to prevent deaths of victims of heart attacks. The decision to integrate medical care in small isolated hospitals with that of an established community hospital, even though it might be located miles away, would appear to be a wise one and is included in the design of the regional system proposed for the United States.

In order to get a regional system off the ground, many a priori decisions will have to be made concerning the distribution of activities in the central, the community, and the cottage hospital. Carefully designed models and simulation studies on the computer will be most helpful in reaching such preliminary decisions. Eventually, after the regional medical program is under way, the exact role of each of these hospitals in the care of the patient will be determined by actual experience and by precisely controlled studies.

Lines of Communication and Transportation within a Regional System

If the regional system is to function as a single institution, the lines of communication and transportation among the constituent hospitals must be definite and flexible and must serve many purposes, including a unified administration, accessibility to effective and acceptable patient care, conservation of professional time, and efficient use of financial, institutional, and technological resources. The elements of interchange include the people served (well and sick), professional personnel, specimens for laboratory examination, information, education, and electronic signals. All of these elements of interchange will depend upon efficient communication and transportation systems which will link all of the constituent hospitals in each region, maintain two-way radio communication with all transporting vehicles, and fan out through the emergency and ambulatory services into the community and to the homes of those cared for in the regional system.

The People Served (Well and Sick)

Each person should be treated insofar as possible by his own physician in his own community hospital. But whenever the maintenance of his health or the prevention and treatment of his disease demand more specialized care, he must be moved to the central hospital. For purposes of efficiency he may have to be moved to another community hospital whose resources—staff, equipment, or organization—are particularly appropriate to the care of his disease.

Many decisions as to the location of care will be relatively easy. Patients needing superspecialists' care and well individuals requiring rare services such as mandatory immunization with perishable vaccines (for example, yellow fever) for foreign travel to certain countries will be cared for in the central hospital. Conversely, following treatment by a superspecialist in the central hospital, if his continuous follow-up supervision is not essential, the patient would be returned to his community hospital for continuing care under the aegis of his personal physician, who would refer him back to the superspecialist when necessary. The treatment of illnesses of intermediate severity will, at first, have to be determined case by case. Eventually, accumulated experience, supported when necessary by computer simulations and finally by field trials, will provide firm guidelines as to location of care.

Other decisions such as the location of intensive and coronary care units may be more difficult. Intensive care is now in fashion. Many hospitals, regardless of function and size, are dashing headlong into the development of intensive and coronary care services, often to the detriment of hospitalized patients not in the special care units. This is so because the high cost of equipment for patients within these units has sometimes limited the availability of funds for the technological support of patients housed elsewhere in the same hospital. High-quality intensive care demands the services of many different kinds of medical specialists and engineers and a large force of allied medical personnel and is fantastically expensive. With efficient transportation and communication in a regional system, it is likely that, except for temporary intensive care for emergencies developing within the community hospital or when geographic considerations dictate otherwise, a higher quality of intensive care for all could be provided if it were concentrated in the central hospital. Control studies on patient outcome and cost effectiveness will be necessary to settle this question. Once again, it must be emphasized that the precise distribution and balance of all medical care resources, including intensive and coronary care units, between central and community hospitals, will depend initially upon decisions based whenever possible on prior knowledge and computer simulation studies and, finally, upon accumulated experience and the results of definitive medical care experiments.

Physicians and Allied Health Personnel
The scarcest asset of medical care is professional time, and everything possible must be done to conserve it. Waste of professional time in moving from place to place must be avoided whenever possible. Other things being equal, the patient and the well person should be moved to the physician and to allied health personnel, rather than vice versa. With a good transportation and communication system, it should take no longer to bring the patient to the doctor than the doctor to the patient. There are, however, situations where the physician or other professional personnel will find it necessary or more efficient to go directly to the patient at his home or in another hospital. For example, the patient's own physician will have to visit him at home whenever he requires

care for an acute episode before he can be moved, or in the central hospital when continuity of care or personal health services become crucial to his recovery. Central hospital consultants in certain specialties, for example, ophthalmology or dermatology, in which consultations on many patients can be conveniently conducted on the same day, will make weekly visits to the community hospital. Emergency consultations in these specialties between the consultant's visits will be provided at the central hospital. The central hospital consultant will also have to provide consultation at the community hospital in certain cases when transportation for the patient is extremely hazardous and when remote measurements via telemetry will not suffice.

The same principle of not wasting professional time in travel applies to allied medical personnel. Care should be provided within the hospital by some allied health personnel such as operating room nurses, laboratory and x-ray technicians, and pharmacists because their services require complex instrumental or other technological resources. The principle is also valid for other specialized allied medical personnel, including pediatric assistants, dietitians, medical social workers, and those in special fields such as neurology and orthopedics.

In contrast, there are medical personnel whose professional duties specifically require that they do home visiting. Travel is essential for the public health nurse or the visiting nurse who performs preventive and therapeutic services. These nurses will be the home visitor in the proposed ambulatory medical care program and, therefore, the key contact point in the local district between the system and the people served. Indeed, a visiting nurse can perform many of the functions that formerly were provided by the physician during a home visit. The nurse visiting in the home will interpret the physician's instructions within the practical limitations of the patient's environment, will reinforce health education of immediate preventive and therapeutic applicability, will administer prescribed injections or collect specimens for laboratory examinations, will identify new health and medical care problems, will supply personal attention, nursing care, reassurance, and comfort to the patient, and will relay information back to the patient's physician. At times for continuity of care she will meet together with the patient and the physician in the hospital. With careful planning, the home visit by the public health nurse may save much professional time for the physician and for other specialized allied medical personnel such as the medical social worker. But, there are times when allied medical personnel, for example, the occupational therapist or a home schoolteacher, may also have to serve a bedridden patient in the home. A careful balance must be struck between medical care needs and the conservation of professional time. Professional time must not be wasted by unnecessary movement from place to place.

Transportation of Laboratory Specimens

Laboratory resources will be divided among the different types of hospitals with the expensive more sophisticated equipment concentrated in the central hospital. As newer physical methods of measurement are developed and adapted for immediate use by the physician—for example, respiratory gas measurements by flowmeter and mass spectrograph—sensors at the bedside will collect and send electrical signals from the patient in the community hospital to a major laboratory installation in the central hospital, where the data will be processed and the results transmitted back to the patient's bedside. Eventually, these physical methods should replace some biochemical methods with their intrinsic limitations. Most biochemical measurements require the collection and processing of specimens, a procedure that introduces all kinds of errors, including loss, breakage, and mix-up of specimens, delays in examination, and failure and mistakes in the reporting of results. But until the physical and engineering sciences yield such technology, most of the frequently needed tests will be performed in automated biochemical and bacteriological laboratories in the community hospital and the uncommon and more demanding tests in the central hospital.

Transportation of specimens for testing should create no great difficulties. The transportation system will be geared for emergency and routine transport of specimens, depending upon the needs of the patient, the nature of the tests, and the perishability of the specimen. The system will be designed to take into account such constraints as time and temperature control on specimen collection, transportation, and testing and on the urgency of the tests results for the management of the patient. Specimens for newly developed, highly specialized, or dangerous tests will, as at present, be shipped elsewhere: to research laboratories in medical schools, to state health department laboratories, or national laboratories such as those at the Center for Disease Control in Atlanta, Georgia.

In very remote areas, as in the cottage hospitals acting as extensions of community hospitals (figure 2), specimen transportation will depend upon the local plan of allocation of medical care responsibilities. Simple tests will be performed locally, and specimens will be transferred to the community or central hospitals for the more complicated tests. But when the patient himself needs more sophisticated management, the specimens will be transmitted within the patient as he is transported for care from the cottage hospital to the community hospital or to the central hospital in the regional care system.

Information Processing 3

If each medical care region is to function as a single institution, the processing of information will have to meet many different needs and act as an integrating force within the region. The needs include individual patient care; clinical research; patient scheduling, alerting, and follow-up; quality control of medical care; administrative operation and efficiency control. Many different types of information will have to be stored, retrieved, and exchanged among all the participating hospitals and other entities such as the emergency control command centers and the district reception centers of the regional care system.

Individual Patient Care

Medical information in records of each individual patient is now spread around among the hospitals, clinics, and doctors' offices where he has previously received preventive or therapeutic services. Essential and even life-saving information may be difficult and, at times, impossible to retrieve.

Medical records are still in a primitive state and reflect the chaos of our unbalanced system of medical care. Although the information in the individual patient record is arranged in some temporal order, the records themselves differ from hospital to hospital and from physician to physician in format, order of presentation of medical, nursing, and other paramedical and laboratory data, and in legibility and the use of abbreviations. Medical record content varies all the way from incomplete lists of high spots of the patient's course to encyclopedic dossiers of information of varying but unknown degrees of reliability, validity, and usefulness. We lack simple standards of reliability and validity of medical record data. There are practically no studies of the relevance of different types and items of medical record information to the maintenance of health and to the prevention and treament of disease. We do nothing about discarding useless and misleading information. Records are bulky and often require hours of time from the physician and other professionals who must review them and miles of shelf space in hospital record rooms. A ray of sunshine, and a good beginning, is the Weed[1] classification of medical record data in accordance with the chief medical problems of the patient.

In the face of all this confusion and with the lack of simple definitions, the elaborate computer processing of

1. L. L. Weed, *Medical Records, Medical Education, and Patient Care: The Problem-Oriented Record as a Basic Tool* (Cleveland: The Press of Case Western Reserve University, 1969).

individual medical records in their present state becomes mere playacting. Much of the data now in hospital records does not deserve to be recorded on paper, let alone to be stored in the memory of the computer. More important, when erroneous clinical information is stored in a computer, the printout with its aura of authenticity may actually mislead the physician and harm the patient. In a word, the confused state of our medical records is merely symptomatic of the way in which medicine itself is now practiced. As an efficient system of medical care is evolved and implemented, the records themselves should become more orderly and, it is to be hoped, more relevant to patient care.

For the medical care of the future and the national health program, we will need a single integrated, reliable, and valid medical record from which the specifically desired information can be retrieved immediately for patient care. The most practical storage unit would be a single central file containing information on all services provided anywhere within the region for each individual resident in each medical care region. Moreover, an interregional record-linkage system should be developed to retrieve information on care given to each person outside of his region of residence for inclusion in his integrated record for continuity of his care and for research purposes.

But we must not wait for the creation of a national health program to develop an integrated patient record. We must ask many questions and perform many studies if we are to have an efficient record system when a national health program becomes operative. What kinds of data are to be recorded and in what detail? How can the reliability and validity of individual items of information be guaranteed? How can we set up separate categories for factual information and interpretive medical reasoning? What is the relative usefulness to the physician and to the patient of individual items of information, such as the result of a particular laboratory test? How can the confidentiality of the record be maintained in the face of the large numbers of physicians and allied medical personnel who will care for the patient? Do we really need to store paper records or could we use disposable computer printouts containing just the information needed to care for the patient during a particular episode or the performance of a specific procedure? These are only a few examples of the problems that must be solved. We must begin now by establishing teams of physicians, statisticians, and engineers in our prestigious hospitals to explore the relevant questions and to develop an integrated, computerized, confidential personal health record system that will store and retrieve exactly the information needed for each individual medical care service and procedure.

When the basic requirements of a computerized record system are met and implemented, patient care will be facilitated and simplified. Thus, on each visit of the patient to his doctor or on admission to a hospital, the patient's physician could retrieve on a paper printout or on an illuminated screen exactly the information needed to provide immediate care. Also, treatment by an allied health professional person, such as a physiotherapist, or a nurse-midwife could be facilitated by a printout of the orders of the physician for the specific episode of care. Preventive medicine can also be made more effective. At each patient visit, the printout could automatically alert the physician to previous undesirable health events that might presage the onset of a preventable or manageable severe illness. For example, the printout could identify a symptom such as bleeding from the bowel that might herald the onset of cancer, the physical finding of a questionably elevated arterial blood pressure that might foretell the evolution of manageable hypertension, or an abnormal test result such as slightly increased eyeball pressure that might be the first manifestation of glaucoma which could lead to blindness. As another example, the immunization schedule of the young infant could be programmed on the computer to alert the physician or pediatric assistant to the particular vaccine to be administered on the day of the well-baby visit. At the end of each medical care episode, the paper record would be discarded and recycled, and the cost of computer operations might be offset by elimination of the enormous expense of paper record storage space and the operation of the hospital record room. A beginning has already been made.[2]

Clinical Research

Retrospective research on clinical records is usually not very rewarding because the data were not originally

2. W. R. Ayers, D. B. Murray, P. Luchsinger, R. E. Snell, and F. G. Burke, "Description of an On-Line Information System for Pediatric Pulmonary Patients. Operational Experiences in the Emergency Rooms of Three Hospitals," *American Review of Respiratory Diseases* 105 (June 1972): pp. 914–919; and Ayers, personal communication (1973).

collected and recorded with the particular study in mind and crucial measurements may be lacking. Nevertheless, a careful systematic review of clinical records may be invaluable for the planning of a prospective study. When patient records are used for clinical research, the confidentiality of the record must be absolute and the patient must not be identified. This objective can be attained if advantage is taken of prior experience with such documents as the confidential birth certificate and with the complete file protection techniques used in defense research. Since it is impossible to anticipate the exact nature of future prospective studies, it is both impractical and wasteful to build up massive collections of clinical data with the hope that somehow they might be useful for future studies. The enormous collaborative study on the etiology of cerebral palsy, mental retardation, and other neurological disorders[3] is the classic example of how large masses of data, blindly collected at great expense, yield relatively little specific information. Instead, for an effective study the research record should consist of the clinical medical records of the patients as the core, supplemented by records and computer programs designed to add just the items of data that are needed to answer the specific questions of the proposed study.

Patient Scheduling
A separate information system using the data in the

3. K. R. Niswander and Myron Gordon, "The Women and Their Pregnancies," *The Collaborative Perinatal Study of the National Institute of Neurological Diseases and Stroke* (Philadelphia: W. B. Saunders, 1972).

single central file will be needed for an appointment system to bring together at the designated place at the proper time the patient, the physician and/or allied medical personnel, and the patient's record including all recent laboratory and other measurements. A computerized tickler file will also be required for the health alerting system (see pp. 232–235); for the scheduling of preventive services such as maternal and child health visits, the immunization of infants, and the screening of individuals susceptible to a particular illness; and for surveillance and follow-up of patients who may be chronically ill or who may be in the early stages of a serious disease.

Administrative Operation

Administrative record keeping in regional medical care has two objectives: to supply the data and interpretation essential for assuring efficient operation of the regional medical system and careful cost control, and to communicate to each category of professional personnel the information needed so that they all may work together effectively. Involved in the first objective is the keeping of a set of books, including management, budget, actuarial, and accounting information, just as is done by a corporation to maintain efficient operation. Indeed, the mere existence of administrative records facilitates the systematic collection of medical information. Thus, in countries where accounting records of individuals in the national health programs exist, for example, the United Kingdom and Sweden, or in voluntary prepayment insurance programs in the United States, the individual financial charges in the cost-accounting records automatically define the nature and date of all medical events and procedures in each patient.

The second objective of administrative record keeping can be attained through an information clearing house, using a phone-book yellow-pages system[4] as an inventory and reference mechanism for identifying and securing the expertise required to perform a specific function. The system should operate effectively if each professional person is completely informed about his own responsibilities and the duties of other personnel with whom he will have to work, and knows how to use the information clearing house whenever additional expertise is needed.

Chapter 13, on the quality control systems, indicates the kind of information that must be collected to measure the efficiency of a medical care system and the quality of care provided to the individuals served by the program.

Professional Education
The professional educational program of a regional system will comprise the undergraduate and postgraduate education of general and specialized physicians under the auspices of the affiliated medical school; qualifying education of allied medical personnel under the direction of local universities and colleges; education at the bedside of the entire "team" of physicians and all allied medical professional personnel that must collaborate if effective and efficient medical care is to be provided to the patient in the central and in the community hospitals of the

4. D. D. Rutstein and Murray Eden, *Engineering and Living Systems: Interfaces and Opportunities* (Cambridge, Massachusetts: MIT Press, 1970): pp. 48 and 52–54.

region; continuing education in collaboration with professional societies of all professional personnel to maintain their competence and keep them abreast of scientific progress; and, through the information clearing house, the instruction necessary to keep all personnel up-to-date on the operation of the medical care system.

In carrying out its fundamental task of relating basic scientific knowledge to clinical medicine, the affiliated medical school in a regional medical care system would have the advantages of the resources of the central hospital for undergraduate and specialist education, the community hospitals for undergraduate education on commonly occurring diseases and for the postgraduate education of the general physician, and the regional system itself for the teaching of the continuity of medical care and of medical prognosis. Comparable advantages from regional organization will accrue to the educational system for allied medical personnel. In essence, with the implementation of a regional system of care, every hospital in every region will be affiliated with a medical school and will become a teaching hospital. This new relationship will demand that new methods of supervisory responsibility within the quality control system will have to be developed to assure that university hospital standards are implemented within every affiliated community hospital.

Allied Medical Professions
Schools of the different allied medical professions are widely scattered and their educational programs are usually not correlated with one another or with medical

education. Thus, at Harvard University, physicians, dentists, and specialists are educated in the medical school and nurses in the affiliated teaching hospitals; public health officers, specialists in public health disciplines, and some allied medical personnel, such as nutritionists and public health nurses, are educated in the school of public health; while other paramedical professions are educated in different schools—for example, medical social workers at Simmons College and physicians' assistants at Northeastern University.

There are two basic requirements for the education of the allied medical professions in the future. The curriculum of each allied medical profession must be based on its defined role in medical care (see chapter 4, "The Medical Manpower Muddle"), and there must be a final common educational pathway so that all concerned with patient care are brought together under university auspices as a team at the patient's bedside for inpatient care and in the clinic for ambulatory medical care.

Electronic Signals
The efficiency of the medical care system will depend on rapid, precise, and directed transfer of information among its units and its personnel. Toward this end, our increasing knowledge of communication networks and technology and their messengers—electronic signals—has a widening spectrum of usefulness in regional systems of care. Demonstrated applications of such a communication system include consultation and primary medical care at a distance, the storage and transmission of medical record information, the control and rapid pro-

cessing of data from laboratory procedures and clinical examinations, the transmission of information in electronic records such as the electrocardiogram, and the implementation of many facets of hospital administration including pharmacy and blood bank inventory, accounting procedures, and management control.

Obvious future applications, in addition to direct measurements on the patient, include the control and implementation of the proposed emergency and ambulatory care programs, the assurance of continuity of individual patient care throughout all the services within the regional system, and the functional interlocking of central and community hospital equipment, personnel, and services to obtain optimal results at lowest possible capital investment and operating costs. Indeed, as medical care increasingly consists of an integrated set of specialized functions, work and flow analyses assume great importance in organizing and operating a medical care system.

A Practical Example: Consultation at a Distance

The future potential of electronic communication in actual medical care can be visualized by an analysis of the task of providing consultation at a distance within a regional system. Much medical time is now wasted by the need, for example, of the consultant to drive, park, and walk as he goes to and from his office to the patient's bedside. Let us examine the possibilities, limitations, and research aspects of substituting electronic signals for the many different kinds of communication usually required for consultation in medical care. The evolution of the required technology is already underway at several sites, including the links between the Massachusetts General Hospital and Logan Airport and the Bedford V. A. Hospital, and in the experiments on medical care consultation in some states, for example, Missouri, Nebraska, and New Hampshire.

Assuming the availability of a well-organized regional system and a competent consultant, two other conditions must be satisfied before effective medical consultation can be provided at a distance. The communication system must be able to transmit the required information, and the medical observations have to be in or be converted into a form that can be transmitted and interpreted effectively at reasonable cost. Both aspects have to be studied in concert to give play to the ingenuity needed to arrive at the trade-offs that could lead to optimal interrelated care.

Let us imagine that in a medical care region a patient in a community hospital requires the services of a consultant located in the central hospital about 45 minutes away by car. The hospitals are linked with the most expensive and the most effective communication system, two-way coaxial cable closed-circuit color television with resolution adequate for interpretation of a chest x-ray, and with color values true enough for recognition in the patient of pallor, flushing, cyanosis, and jaundice. The consultant will thus be trading off immediate access to the patient—that is, being able to touch him—for the saving of the hour and a half of his time (about one-sixth of his working day) that he would lose in traveling.

Consultation at a Distance

The consultant goes to the studio in the central hospital and greets, on the screen, his patient lying in bed, with his doctor and a nurse-technician at his bedside. The patient's physician states the chief complaint and briefly summarizes the present illness and the past history of the patient. The consultant then rounds out the history by obtaining answers to questions directed to the physician and to the patient.

The patient's physician then demonstrates, on the screen, significant findings in the physical examination, including the appearance of the patient, skin lesions, paralysis, limitations in movement, disturbances in breathing, areas of tenderness and swelling, and abnormal reflexes. The nurse-technician will place the microphone of the electronic stethoscope at those places where the consultant may hear, through the earpieces in the studio in the central hospital, the abnormal sounds that had suggested to the patient's physician either lung dysfunction or disturbed heart action. The consultant may also wish to listen at certain spots on the chest which he will identify by verbal instructions and by a remote-controlled spotlight. The physician or nurse would then place the microphone sequentially on the selected spots as the consultant completes his examination of the chest. At the end of the patient's personal physician's demonstration of his positive findings on physical examination, he will, upon request, elicit other physical findings of specific interest to the consultant. During the consultation, the quantitative results of laboratory tests may be flashed on the screen, x-ray films may be viewed directly, and electronic records such as those of the electrocardiogram and electroencephalogram may be read and interpreted.

The results of such a consultation at a distance will often provide the basis for a decision to transfer the patient to the central hospital where other procedures could be performed, or for reassurance to the patient that he is doing well and nothing further needs to be done. The consultation would then have accomplished its purpose. But in order to increase the probability of successful consultations at a distance in the future, let us explore the development of new technology for this purpose.

All of the above procedures have depended on the transfer of either visual or auditory information from the patient and his attendants to the eyes and ears of the consultant. These methods of communication will have to be carefully explored because the structure and lighting of the color television studio can either facilitate or obstruct the examination of the patient. For example, Dr. Charles Sanders and I examined two patients with chronic severe liver disease over the Massachusetts General Hospital–Bedford Veterans Administration Hospital television link, and were impressed with how healthy the patients looked after almost a decade of illness. When we drove out to Bedford immediately afterward for direct examination of the same patients, we were surprised because they both looked very sick. We discovered that the lighting in the televisions studio at Bedford was designed, as in the case of most television studios, to "make everybody look good." This policy may work well for TV entertainers, for for precise clinical examination, television lighting will have to be changed to make people look the way they are. On the other hand, over the same television link, the spacious view and the bright lighting on the patient permitted us to make observations that would have been very difficult on direct examination. It was, for example, easy to measure the excursion of the diaphragm by watching the ripple of the muscles on the side of the chest as the diaphragm moved up and down with each breath—an observation that is very difficult for the physician to make at the patient's bedside.

Additional technology must also be developed to facilitate the visual examination of the patient at a distance. For example, within the next few years it should be possible to examine the interior of orifices of the human body by visual inspection at a distance. The technology already exists for the development of instruments taking advantage of fibro-optics for visual examination of the interior of the mouth, throat, nose, eyes, ears, rectum, bladder, and female genitalia. Some instruments for such purposes are already available, but much work remains to be done to produce all of them at reasonable cost and to interlock them with the telemetry of a television system.

The greatest obstacle to examination at a distance is the need for the consultant in "the laying on of hands" to depend on his sense of touch during his examination of the patient. But even here technology can be useful. For example, an instrument has been developed to transmit vibrations such as those a physician might feel when he places his hand on the chest of a patient suffering from the kind of heart disease that obstructs the flow of blood or from pneumonia, when the inflamed surface (pleura) of the lung scrapes against the chest wall. That instrument is now being used in medical teaching to transmit abnormal vibrations from the chest of the patient to the hands of medical students as they remain in their seats in the amphitheater during the presentation of the patient. It could be modified to transmit either cardiac vibrations or pleural rubs from the patient in the community hospital to the consultant in the central hospital.

It might also become possible by the development of new technology from existing scientific knowledge to estimate at a distance the size of the solid organs in the abdomen—the liver, spleen, and kidneys—a procedure that is now manually performed by the physician at the bedside. It is theoretically possible that by measuring the degree of interference to the passage of ultrasound waves through the abdomen one could estimate the size of the solid organs within that cavity.

This last example leads to a basic principle in the development of techniques from scientific knowledge for examination of a patient at a distance. The instruments should not be designed to imitate what the physician would do if he were with the patient. The physician now obtains information on the size of the liver, for example, by percussion of the right lower chest and palpation of the upper abdomen. It would obviously be silly to try to imitate the physician and build a robot to place its mechanical hand on the right upper abdomen of the patient to feel for an enlarged liver. Instead, the question is, How can technology be developed to provide the physician with the information he needs to evaluate his patient at a distance?

Unfortunately, it is unlikely that instruments will be developed that will permit a physician to conduct at a distance most of the procedures that depend upon his sense of touch at the bedside of the patient. Examples are the detection of irregularities of the skull and other bones, abnormal but invisible soft-tissue masses, enlargement of the lymph glands, the "surgical examination" of the abdomen, and manual examination of the orifices of the body, including the rectum and the vagina. But these obstacles may not be insuperable.

What is the purpose of consultation at a distance? Ideally, consultations should yield a definitive diagnosis and course of treatment. But, practically speaking, the purpose of consultation at a distance in a regional system of care would be well served by the decision as to whether the patient's condition requires transportation to the central hospital or whether he can be treated effectively in the community hospital. This decision can probably be made in practically all cases using only the observations that existing technology makes possible. If the patient is so seriously ill that he has to be moved to the central hospital, any desired examination procedure can be performed by the consultant after transfer of the patient. If, on the contrary, examination at a distance reveals that the patient is well enough to be managed easily in his own hospital, the purpose of the consultation would also have been served. For the very few patients who are not obviously sick enough to require transfer and yet not well enough for simple treatment, and where consultative examinations that cannot now be performed at a distance are crucial to the locus of patient management, it may be necessary for the consultant to make a visit to the patient or to employ specially trained supertechnicians to aid his general physician to obtain the information that would have been yielded by a specialist's examination at the bedside.

Methods of Communication for Consultation within a Regional System

It is clear that with closed-circuit color television in a regional system many essentials of medical consultation at a distance could be satisfied and much physician's time could be saved. But closed-circuit coaxial cable color television is very expensive; in fact, it is too expensive for nationwide use in regional medical care. However, when such technology cannot be made available and cannot be financed, more limited consultation can be performed with simpler methods of communication. These are slow-scan television, picture and sound transmission over telephone lines, or sound transmission alone over the telephone.

Slow-scan television yields an interrupted series of still pictures instead of continuous motion and does not require a coaxial cable network. It, therefore, permits sharply focused still pictures of the patient but not of his movements. Nevertheless, this method does have many practical uses. For example, the appearance of the patient's face, the details of a skin rash, the image of an x-ray film, and the appearance of blood cells or bacteria under the microscope could all be viewed at a distance.

A system has been developed in the Bell Laboratories for transmission of a black and white image of the person at the other end of the telephone line. The Picturephone does permit observation of a patient and his movements, but the resolution is so relatively poor that, for example, an x-ray of the chest could not be interpreted at a distance. However, if the rate of transmission over telephone lines were slowed down to give a series of still pictures, as in slow-scan television, resolution would improve. With a switching device, it would then be possible either to view a relatively hazy picture of the patient's movements or to see the fine details of an x-ray film in a series of still pictures. Thus, this method now under study[5] might meet some of the needs of a physician practicing medicine at a distance.

Sound transmission alone over the telephone, as at present, has distinct but limited usefulness. The consultant may answer specific questions raised by the physician or the patient over the telephone; but when he does so, he makes the assumption that the observations upon which the questions are based are both valid and reliable. Since he cannot see the patient, his appraisal may be completely inaccurate. This conclusion is documented by the oft-repeated experience of every consultant, who, having heard the history of a patient in an adjoining room, is led into the bedchamber and may be shocked by

5. C. D. Stockbridge, "The Performance of Picturephone[(R)] Systems in Transmitting Medical Data," in *Application of Optical Instrumentation in Medicine*, Proceedings of the Society of Photo-Optical Instrumentation Engineers Symposium (Chicago, 1972).

the difference between his mental image and the actual appearance of the patient. Nevertheless, once the consultant has seen the patient, the telephone may provide for excellent communication between the consultant and the patient's physician.

Much research and development must be done in exploring and defining the relative usefulness of each of these methods of communication in a regional system of medical care. The reward would be the saving of much professional time which eventually will be translated into a need for a smaller total number of physicians.

The communications system for consultation at a distance in a regional medical program must also provide another essential ingredient of all medical consultation. It must permit the consultant and the physician to discuss the case out of earshot of the patient, so that they may be able to weld their professional knowledge calmly and objectively into a clear-cut course of action for the most effective treatment of the disease, for building the morale of the patient, and for clarifying the situation to the family.

The Region: The Operating Unit for Medical Care

Each region will be the operating unit for medical care and will represent a medical service area with a population of one to three million people. The size, shape, and boundaries of each region will depend upon such factors as the placement of the central and community hospitals, population groupings, geographical characteristics, the location of industrial and shopping centers, the flow patterns of highways and other methods of transporta-

The Region: Operating Unit for Medical Care

tion, and the lines of communication. Whenever possible, the functional center of each region will be a medical school affiliated hospital. The boundaries of each medical care region may but will not always coincide with state or municipal boundaries. Thus, western Massachusetts might have Albany, New York, as its regional focus, while northern Indiana might be served by a medical school in Chicago, Illinois.

Metropolitan areas where more than one medical school exist would be divided into a group of regions, each with its own central hospital, which would fan out to cover the surrounding areas. In Boston, for example, the Massachusetts General Hospital could serve the north shore of Massachusetts to the New Hampshire boundary line; the Harvard Medical School hospital complex would be the focus for the region northwest and west of Boston; the Boston University Medical Center would be the central hospital for the area to the south and southwest of Boston; and the Tufts University Medical Center would be the focal point for the south shore of Massachusetts and be within helicopter range of the tip of Cape Cod. The region of southern Massachusetts and adjacent Cape Cod would be well served by the teaching hospitals affiliated with Brown University Medical School in Providence, Rhode Island.

In metropolitan areas where two or more regions coexist, not every central hospital would provide every superspecialist service. The location of the more uncommon services would depend on the relative resources of the different central hospitals. Thus, congenital heart surgery could be concentrated in one of the central hospitals, while the highly specialized peripheral nerve surgery essential to sewing back a limb that has been accidentally amputated, might be performed in another central hospital in the same metropolitan area.

The central hospital of each medical care region will be the focus of decentralization for the national medical care program at the same time that it serves as the focus of centralization for its own region. Quality control procedures, national professional standards, health indices, and priorities emanating from the Federal Health Board (chapter 14) will be implemented in each region through the regional health board (pp. 207–208). At the same time, the statistical data in the guidance system (chapter 13) collected by the National Center for Health Statistics, and the epidemiological observations in the early warning system by the Center for Disease Control (chapter 13) will be used to evaluate the effectiveness of medical care in the region. The information would then be fed back to the national program for comparative analysis of regional health, the improvement of standards, the creation of health indices, and the establishment of priorities of health and medical care services.

Within each region, and in accordance with recommendations of the Federal Health Board, professional standards and indices, scientific knowledge, medical communication, transportation technology, and general and specialized medical and allied health services will flow centrifugally from the central to the community hospitals. In turn, the area served by each community hospital will be divided into districts, each of which will have its own ambulatory care program tied into the

Figure 3. Ambulatory care.

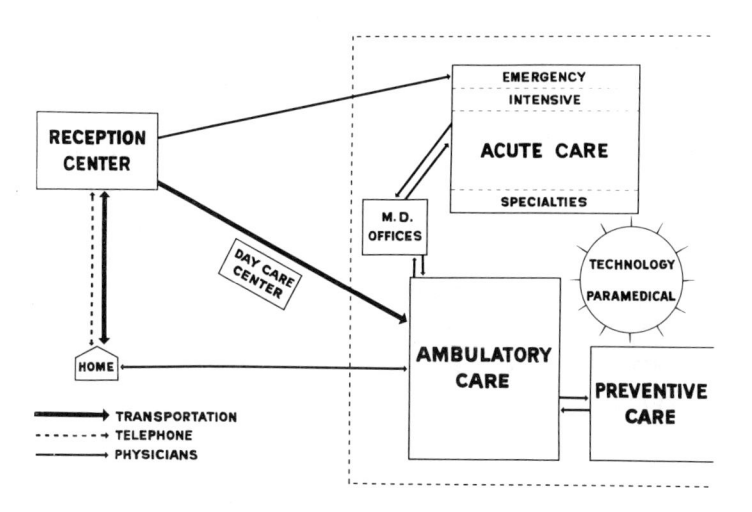

community hospital (chapter 7 and figure 3). In each district, there will be a health committee representing the residents of its community and responsible for calling attention to the special needs created by the cultural, economic, geographic, and population characteristics of the area served. Thus, the centrifugal flow of scientific and professional knowledge from the central to the community hospitals would be carefully interwoven with the centripetal flow of information defining the needs of each small community in the region.

At the time of inauguration of the local medical care program, there will be individuals and families who have well-established and often cherished arrangements for their medical care. Every effort will have to be made to continue such practice with gradual change as time goes on, as the older generation dies off, and as needs arise that are better served by the district program.

In this blueprint, administration and quality control of the proposed health services would encompass the potential benefit of the medical services, the professional care technology, and the special needs of the population served in order that the professional, institutional, economic, personnel, and social resources of the region may be used to their fullest extent. The education of the physician and allied health personnel will also be facilitated by the regional structure. Indeed, the recommended uniform structure of regional medical care makes unnecessary the bifid program of university health science centers and health education centers recommended by the Carnegie Commission on Higher Education.[6] Finally, each medical care region will provide an excellent population unit for research on medicine and medical care delivery. In a word, the medical care regional system focused on a medical school teaching hospital will, at one and the same time, serve as an effective base for medical care, for education, and for research.

It may be concluded that an appropriately designed regional medical care system can make possible a higher quality of medical care for all of the people, conserve the time of the physician and of allied health personnel, and diminish the demand for hospital beds which, in turn,

6. The Carnegie Commission on Higher Education, *Higher Education and the Nation's Health. Policies for Medical and Dental Education. A Special Report and Recommendations* (New York: McGraw-Hill, 1970).

will decrease both capital investment and operating costs. Most important of all, the proposed regional system would identify and interrelate all of the medical care resources, and define and repair the gaps in care, and thereby provide the institutional structure within which every person could receive the kind of medical care that he needs when he needs it.

The Medical Manpower Muddle 4

The confused state of American medical care is compounded by the medical manpower muddle. The tasks for which each category of medical manpower is responsible are undefined, depend upon tradition and local custom, and vary widely throughout the country. Each profession through its own organizations, for example, the American Medical Association, the American Nurses Association, and the American Society of Medical Technologists, stakes out its independent area of professional activity usually without consultation with representatives of other closely related professional medical groups.

State licensure laws do qualify physicians and allied medical personnel to practice their professions. These laws, whether or not they take advantage of the voluntary qualifying examinations of the National Board of Medical Examiners, vary from state to state. The state licensure laws do establish minimal requirements for each of the professions in order to exclude quacks and charlatans but they do not qualify professionally trained persons to perform in defined roles. Most state laws licensing physicians give broad overall approval to every qualified Doctor of Medicine to practice any aspect of his profession. Thus, a qualified physician may be a general practitioner or may practice in any specialty of medicine from pediatrics to neurosurgery regardless of his aptitude, education, training, or experience. The national specialty boards have established standards for specialists and do accept responsibility for their qualification but they have no official status. In summary, it is clear that our licensure laws are not uniform, are antiquated, and are not being updated to satisfy the requirements of modern medical care.

There is a great imbalance between the broad authority given to the physician by state licensure laws and the narrow restrictions limiting the activities of the allied medical professions. The imbalance has probably evolved from the physician's fear that members of the allied medical professions might "practice medicine." To be sure, the physician as captain of the medical team must be completely aware of the contributions of each kind of paramedical professional so that he may be able to interrelate individual activities for the benefit of the patient. But, when the physician himself performs tasks that do not demand his knowledge, background, education, and experience, he wastes our scarcest medical care asset—the physician's time. Physicians should prescribe, but should not be occupied with the more routine mechanical tasks such as intravenous therapy, lumbar puncture, insertion of tubes into the windpipe, application of splints, administration of vaccines, and the standardized segments of major and minor surgical procedures. Many of these tasks can be performed better by specially trained supertechnicians than by the average physician.

To compensate for the imbalance between the scope of licensure of the physician and of the other medical professions, the laws tend to be violated when, under the guise of medical supervision, allied health personnel perform tasks in which they may have become competent but which are beyond their legal authority. A classic example is the nurse in the coronary care unit who, without any immediate medical supervision, has to make on-the-spot life and death decisions such as the selection and dosage of powerful drugs when the patient suddenly develops an irregularity of the heartbeat that may threaten his life. To correct the imbalance, the licensure laws should define more precisely the various roles of the physician and should expand the authority of the allied medical professions to perform the tasks for which they have been qualified and which do not demand the total competence of the physician.

We are in a muddle because the lack of precise definition of the individual tasks to be performed by each category of medical manpower has resulted in overlapping functions on the one hand and gaps in services on the other. Overlapping functions result when professional personnel perform technical services, and technicians assume professional responsibilities, or when a specialty of one of the professions is created at the boundary line of another profession. Thus, the medically qualified ophthalmologist wastes his time in routine testing of eyes for eyeglasses, while the technically trained optometrist, referred to in some states as "doctor," may at times overinterpret his findings in the form of a diagnosis. The boundary between nursing and social work has been obscured by the creation of public health nurses by the one profession and medical social workers by the other. The public health nurse and the medical social worker tend to stumble over each other in carrying out their missions, with the former having a wider scope of activity in rural areas, and the latter in urban areas. Actually, in the case of these two professions, if the tasks to be performed and the educational programs were clearly defined, one individual with consultative advice from both sides could be educated to carry the responsibility now allocated separately to the two professions.

In the meantime, major gaps in services remain unfilled. Our unnecessarily high infant mortality rates are partly due to the lack of nurse-midwives to care for normal pregnancies and perform normal deliveries under the supervision of a physician who could then spend his time where it is most needed, that is, to provide intensive care to high-risk patients. Similarly, the failure to define manpower requirements for emergency care—for example, the medical qualifications of the driver of an emergency vehicle—obstructs efforts to decrease our excessive death rates from highway accidents.

Newer categories of allied medical personnel are being created without any systematic comparative analysis of their tasks with those already being performed by members of existing medical professions. Inevitably, this process leads to wasteful duplication of services with ever-growing interprofessional rivalries. The most recent example is the introduction of military medical corpsmen as physicians' assistants in civilian medical care. Although there is an urgent need for the services of medical military corpsmen in civilian emergency care systems and in the manning of ambulances and other medical transportation vehicles, many of their newly assigned duties as physicians' assistants merely duplicate those now being performed by nurses. The American Nurses Association has already violently reacted. The inefficiency, wastefulness, excessive costs, and jurisdictional strikes that result from such parallel catch-as-catch-can evolution among workers in parallel fields has been amply demonstrated in the history of the building trades. If present trends continue, that unhappy history will be repeated by the allied medical professions. In both groups of occupations, tasks are defined in terms of the scope of activity of each of the individual vocations, rather than the most effective performance of the defined procedure. For the future, we can plan and operate a system of medical care in which the roles of the individual medical and allied medical professions are not ends in themselves but become subservient to the patient's need for preventive, curative, and life-saving services.

In the face of a situation where both the system of operation and the individual roles of the participants remain undefined, it is difficult to understand how anyone could make any reliable estimates of medical manpower to satisfy future needs. The President's Manpower Commission in 1967 did point up the difficulty of making estimates without definitions although three years later estimates were published in the Carnegie Commission Report.[1]

Actually, if medical care remains in its present chaotic state, there simply will never be enough physicians, nurses, or other medical personnel to do the job. Physicians will continue to be overconcentrated in suburban areas and will be impossible to find in the jungles of our large cities and in our wide open rural spaces. General physician services will become ever more scarce. Some medical specialties such as radiation therapy, neurosurgery, and general surgery will continue to grow far beyond the need for such services. This situation results from financial incentives and the need for highly trained resident physicians who in a very short time are ready to move on to services of their own. Moreover, if psychiatrists continue to limit their practice to a few patients with relatively minor psychiatric disease, there never will be enough of them even if all of the increasing numbers of graduates of all of our medical schools become members of that one specialty.

The same wasteful situation exists among the allied medical professions. although progress has been made in a few areas. For example, during the past decade, the introduction of intensive care and coronary care units has more effectively allocated nursing time for seriously ill

1. The Carnegie Commission on Higher Education, *Higher Education and the Nation's Health. Policies for Medical and Dental Education. A Special Report and Recommendations* (New York: McGraw-Hill, 1970).

patients. But, elsewhere, we continue to waste nursing time by the routine one-to-one allocation of private duty nurses to individual patients while many chronic care institutions responsible for many patients do not have a single nurse on night duty. Unless we work out more efficient ways of allocating nursing time among all of the patients who need it, we will never educate enough nurses to meet future needs.

The Solution of the Manpower Muddle

The solution of the medical manpower muddle demands a series of precise studies of the role performed by each of the professions by identifying the actual tasks now performed by them. With such information, it would be possible to reallocate tasks in order to do away with duplication, to avoid gaps in service, and to be sure that the profession and its tasks are appropriate to each other. The studies of current tasks would be conducted first on physicians in their various professional categories and then on each of the allied medical professions.

Let us use the study of the role of physicians in medical care as an example. The first step is the listing of the tasks actually being performed on an average day by random samples of general physicians and of each category of medical specialist. The list of tasks so collected would be divided into two categories: those which demand the knowledge, background, education, and experience of the physician, and those which do not. For example, in well-baby clinics a neurological examination, if required, would have to be done by a physician, while an estimate of the stage of the baby's development could be made by a trained pediatric assistant. The tasks not requiring the competence of the physician would then be divided into two groups: those that should be performed by the physician himself because each is an important step in the workup and total management of the patient; and those that should be transferred to a particular allied medical profession, to a technological device, or to both. The results of these studies would guide the allocation of appropriate tasks to the physician and to each category of allied medical personnel and would provide estimates of the amount of physician's time that could be salvaged for the duties and responsibilities that really do require his competence. Although this approach may appear to be idealistic, it would be interesting to see the results of the studies and examine the possibilities of their practical implementation.

This same kind of study, analysis, and reallocation of tasks would be conducted for each of the allied medical professions. Subsequently, it would be possible to identify duplications and gaps in service for all of the medical and allied health professions, and the amount of professional time that could be saved in each category.

Eventually, this process should yield precise definitions of the role of the physician and that of each of the allied health professions. In turn, it should lead to the education of a smaller proportion of physicians and of the higher salaried allied health personnel, and to the education and training of a larger proportion of allied health personnel with fewer educational qualifications. This shifting of tasks among the health professions should decrease the total cost of health personnel and the total time and expense of their education. To be sure, it is always difficult to change obsolete patterns of professional activity. But the continuing exponential rise in medical care costs will force the issue. The availability of solid data and a plan for the more effective use of all medical personnel should carry much weight. Fortunately, studies of this kind are already underway at the University of Wisconsin[2] and at the Naval Medical Research Institute at Bethesda, Maryland, where they are being implemented in the allocation of appropriate tasks to medical corpsmen in the United States Navy.[3]

The data yielded by the proposed task studies would also make it possible for the first time to design curricula for the education of all kinds of physicians that would be directly relevant to their future roles. Indeed, to reach that objective there is outlined in this blueprint in detail a structure of a multichannel medical curriculum (chapter 11). The results of the proposed studies could guide the selection of the content of each curricular pathway to include the practical procedures as well as the knowledge of the basic sciences that the physician must have for a complete and thorough understanding of the principles of patient care in the prevention and treatment of illness for which he is responsible. If the same process were followed for each of the allied medical professions, curricula could

2. F. L. Golloday, M. F. Hansen, J. H. Renner, and K. R. Smith, "A Protocol for Study of Health Manpower in Ambulatory Care Practice," Research Report Series, no. 22, University of Wisconsin Health Economics Research Center (December 1972).
3. O. C. Upchurch, "A System Model for the Education and Training of Health Care Delivery Personnel," presented at the American Association for the Advancement of Science Symposium (December 26, 1972).

be developed that would be directly relevant to the specific role of each of them.

If we combine this blueprint of a medical care plan with the redefined roles of medical and paramedical personnel and a set of priorities of medical care objectives and a regional medical system focused on university teaching hospitals, relatively precise estimates could be made of the numbers needed of each of the categories of medical personnel. We could then cease the practice of meeting every medical care crisis by blindly creating new kinds of medical personnel or by constantly increasing the number of physicians, nurses, and other existing categories of medical manpower. Clearing up the medical manpower muddle and a periodic review of professional tasks performed by each of the professions could place the estimates of the number required in each category and the recruitment and education of medical personnel on an objective, logical, and feasible basis. We must have clear-cut medical manpower policies if we are to have effective and efficient medical care.

Emergency Medical Care: The First Step

5

With the institutional structure of regional medical care and a proposed solution to the medical manpower problem as background, let us begin to assemble the functioning elements as modules of a national medical care program. We find that at present two essential elements—emergency and ambulatory medical care— are in a completely chaotic state. To fill these gaps we must, therefore, propose specific programs in both of these areas before a blueprint of a national program can be drawn.

There are many advantages in instituting an emergency care system as the first step in a total program.[1] Many of the elements of emergency care such as the communications system will supply the underpinnings for ambulatory care. Emergency care is relatively easy to

1. D. D. Rutstein, "The Coming Revolution in Medicine: A New Plan for Ambulatory Medical Care," in *Mainstreams of Medicine*, ed. L. S. King (Austin: University of Texas Press, 1971): pp. 74–89.

implement and is not overly expensive. The care of emergencies has been peripheral to the mainstream of current medical practice and its systemization is not likely to precipitate a major conflict with the medical profession. The objectives and accomplishments of emergency care are clear-cut and easy to evaluate. The saving of life in emergencies is so dramatic that it will be relatively simple to demonstrate to physicians and to the public the advantages of a systematic approach to medical care. Above all, in the introduction of a new system of ambulatory care, we must be sure that no patient is harmed in the process of changeover. A smoothly operating emergency care program would assure the effective treatment of life-threatening medical and surgical events which would make it possible to take a more thoughtful, unhurried, and thoroughgoing approach to the design and implementation of an efficient ambulatory program in a complete medical care system.

The sine qua non of a medical and surgical emergency care program is smooth, continuous operation without loss of time from the moment of injury until everything possible has been done for the patient, followed by a directed effort to prevent similar incidents in the future. The mechanism of the reporting of each emergency and the response of the system to it must be efficient. The patient must be kept alive, and if possible, his condition improved during the shortest possible transportation time to the treatment center where resources are available to give him immediate, complete, and effective treatment. The lessons learned from each accident must be fitted into the program to try to prevent similar emergencies in the future.

Instead of a smoothly operating emergency care system, emergency care in most of the United States now usually consists of a disjointed, interrupted series of events without complete integration from moment of injury to effective treatment. The public is poorly informed about how to secure help in an emergency. When there is communication between the emergency case and the treatment center, it tends to be casual. Transportation may be hit-or-miss. The emergency vehicle is rarely manned with personnel trained to care for the patient during transportation. Each medical and surgical emergency station operates in its own self-centered way and because of a lack of a warning system may not be able to plan for the care of a particular emergency case until it appears upon the doorstep. Haphazard distribution and disorganized operation of emergency stations may result in the loss of precious time as a patient is shifted from hospital to hospital in search of necessary specialized care. Witness the delay in the treatment of the late Senator Robert F. Kennedy in Los Angeles when, with a bullet in his brain, he was rushed to a hospital that was unable to care for him. He had then to be transferred to another hospital equipped and staffed to cope with brain injuries. As events proved, the loss of time in his treatment probably made no difference in the outcome, but in some cases unnecessary delay and disorganization will make the difference between life and death.

There is, however, a growing recognition that better emergency care is sorely needed. The National Academy of Sciences has established standards for ambulance design and the training of emergency care personnel.[2] The Department of Health, Education, and Welfare has set up a few test areas where emergency care is being explored. Throughout the country and taking advantage of public interest growing out of publicity following major catastrophes and the fascination with dramatic gadgets, many individual elements of emergency care are being designed and implemented. For example, trauma services are being evolved, "heartmobiles" have been designed for transportation of heart attack victims, poison control centers have been established, hospitals are operating helicopter transportation units, practicing physicians have organized into emergency teams, and discharged military medical corpsmen are being employed for emergency care. All of these efforts are praiseworthy and promising, but to be truly effective they must be interrelated into a smoothly operating program in which the individual segments, each of whose effectiveness has been documented by careful study, are fitted together and contribute efficiently to the immediate care of the patient.

Since the armed forces have had the greatest success in the treatment of emergency casualties, we will call upon their experience in proposing a model of civilian emergency medical care. It has often been said that a soldier in Vietnam received far more effective emergency care

2. Committee on Emergency Medical Services, Division of Medical Sciences, "Roles and Resources of Federal Agencies in Support of Comprehensive Emergency Medical Services," National Academy of Sciences–National Research Council (March 1972).

than an injured civilian on a modern American superhighway. That statement was documented by the constant improvement in the recovery rate among battlefield casualties in contrast with the relatively unchanging rate of civilian auto accident fatalities.

The Military Experience in Emergency Care
The military experience has demonstrated the value of six interrelated essential elements, all of which are lacking in most civilian emergency services. The essentials are:
1. a single director with authority and responsibility;
2. an areawide program that takes advantage of all available medical resources;
3. a communication system that interrelates through a control command center with
4. a transportation system geared to meet geographic and strategic needs and manned by
5. paramedical assistants (corpsmen) specifically trained for on-the-spot care and triage[3] of battle casualties; and
6. a series of emergency care centers each specifically designed and appropriately staffed to treat defined medical and surgical problems.

The experience in Vietnam demonstrated that a program of first-aid care by a corpsman in the front lines

3. This word, coming into civilian use, is an adaptation of the military term that denotes the process by which injured soldiers are sorted out on the battlefield for transfer to the most appropriate medical care facility. It must be clear that triage is not diagnosis. It is the process of making decisions as to the kind of treatment needed by the patient and the type of facilities to which he should then be referred.

with transportation of the casualties to a fully equipped and staffed hospital, yielded better results than care by a battalion surgeon in the front lines. With efficient communication and a medical corpsman to provide on-the-spot first-aid, resuscitation, splinting, intravenous treatment, and reassurance, followed by rapid transportation to the emergency treatment center, the military patient is cared for in the hospital behind the lines by a physician who has at hand the benefits of technological, medical, paramedical, and specialists' support—that is, all the essential constituents of modern emergency medical care.

A Regional Emergency Program

Let us transfer the six essential elements of military emergency care to civilian life in the proposed regional medical care program. First, a physician must be appointed medical director and be given the authority and responsibility for the medical operation of the entire emergency system, including its medical services. Under the aegis of the regional medical officer (pp. 251–252) and with the help of a professional advisory committee, he will be responsible for the implementation of the medical standards of the program, working through the director of each individual hospital emergency station and by collaboration with the communication controller and the transportation coordinator.

The physician-director, or a member of his staff, will be on duty or on call twenty-four hours a day for guidance of the triage nurse in the control center, for supervision of the emergency aides (corpsmen) in the field, and for advice to individual emergency stations on the special preparations needed for unusual casualties being referred to them. In any major catastrophe, the physician-director will supervise the coordination of emergency medical care activities and the emergency medical team either at the command center or at the site of the emergency.

Next, the program should serve the entire regional medical service area, that is, it should be coterminus with the region to be served in the total medical care program. Fragmentation, as at present, along institutional and political lines results in the ineffective use of essential specialized resources and personnel. In most metropolitan areas each separate community has its own emergency service, with the result that there is a wasteful multiplication of capital expenditures for emergency vehicles, care stations, and medical equipment. As a result, operating costs are inflated and personnel are not effectively used. More important, not every community can supply all of the specialized resources demanded by every medical emergency. Witness an accident in Cambridge, Massachusetts, when a child had his eye perforated by a point of a sharp stick wielded by his playmate. A physician who saw the incident called the fire department, the agency locally responsible for ambulance service, and an ambulance promptly appeared. The physician requested the driver to transport the patient to the Massachusetts Eye and Ear Infirmary, an institution world renowned for the quality of its eye surgery, located in Boston on the Charles River just at the other end of the bridge from Cambridge. The driver regretfully refused because of instructions that all emergency cases in Cambridge are to be treated in the nearest Cambridge hospital. A telephone call from the physician to the fire department finally set matters right in this particular case. But the incident dramatized the need for an areawide regional emergency care system if each patient is to receive the benefits of all available medical resources.

The Emergency Communications Network

The integrating force of an emergency medical program is a comprehensive communications network flowing into a communications command center. Later, when the emergency care program is integrated within a regional total care system, the function of the command center in the network will be expanded to implement ambulatory care and to coordinate it with all of the other activities that constitute total medical care.

The communications network must include every telephone in the local system, including household telephones; pay telephones where emergency calls may be made without the use of a coin by dialing the special number of the regional system; the communications posts in police cars, ambulances, fire apparatus, taxis, and common carriers; the "walkie-talkie" phones in emergency vehicles; and the telephones in subsidiary command centers, such as each of the emergency stations in the participating hospitals and the reception center in each ambulatory care district (chapter 6). Emergency phones must be placed along the highways, in poverty areas, and at industrial and other sites where accidents or emergency medical illnesses are likely to be frequent. Highway mileposts (similar to those in European countries, where every tenth of a kilometer is marked) will be needed for the precise geographic location of accident victims. A signaling system for passing motorists will have to be created. A public education program on personal injury and accident reporting will have to be instituted, conducted, and tested. Emphasis must be placed on the need for immediate and precise reporting to assure early treatment. Moreover, the public must understand the danger to individuals and to the entire community created by false alarms and trivial complaints that may clog the network.

The command communication center will be manned for medical triage by public health nurses backed up by a physician on call, transportation experts to supervise the maintenance, deployment, and operation of the emergency vehicles, and a communications engineer and telephone operators to assure efficient network operation around the clock.

Each incoming and medical emergency call will be referred to the triage nurse who will classify the patient by severity, select the emergency station, if any, to which the patient is to be transported, and determine whether the condition of the patient demands special handling during transportation. In studies performed in the Family Health Program of the Massachusetts General Hospital in the 1950s, it was demonstrated that a specially trained public health nurse with access when needed to a physician's advice on the same telephone extension can evaluate medical and surgical problems and perform effective triage. Actually, the public health nurse made one of three decisions: (1) the patient was so sick that he required medical care by a physician, either immediately or by appointment; or (2) the patient was so well that a physician's services were not needed and first aid or simple advice solved his problem; or (3) the nurse was not able to make a decision, at which time (about once in every fifteen calls) she obtained advice and guidance from the physician. For that experience, it is likely that with special training in medical and surgical emergency care a nurse may perform effective triage in an emergency care system.

Whenever a decision is made to transport a patient to an emergency care station, the triage nurse will communicate with the nurse in charge of that facility, who will deploy physicians and allied medical personnel and all necessary equipment and supplies in anticipation of the arrival of the patient.

The Transportation System

The transportation system comprises the services of all emergency vehicles under the control and supervision of the transportation coordinator in the command center. All kinds of vehicles including ambulances, helicopters, first-aid cars, taxis, private cars, and common carriers are necessary to the emergency program. The standard vehicle is the ambulance used for patients whose condition demands transportation in the horizontal position under the care of an emergency aide in an area where highway transportation is adequate. The number, garage location, and deployment of the ambulances in the program will depend on an analysis of the population served, and of the local geographic distribution of medical and surgical emergencies and of treatment centers, and on the flow patterns between them.

Working under the general supervision of the medical director and cooperatively with the triage nurse, the transportation coordinator must be able to relate the particular medical or surgical emergency to the appropriate emergency vehicle and understand the reasons for referral for treatment to a specific emergency center. The drivers and operators of the emergency vehicles are under his direct supervision.

During transportation, certain categories of patients will require immediate treatment or medical supervision. It is not necessary or desirable to man each emergency vehicle with a physician. Instead, borrowing from the military experience, there is a need for a new allied health assistant whom we shall call "emergency aide." At the moment, his qualifications would be those of a discharged military corpsman with experience in the handling of military casualties, with special training in the management of medical emergencies, and reoriented so that he may provide his services in the framework of civilian medical care. The emergency aide must be able to perform first aid and resuscitation; administer intravenous treatment; manage life-threatening irregularities of rhythm following heart attacks with drugs or, if necessary, with a defibrillator; apply a splint to a fracture; perform a normal delivery and free the airway of a newborn baby; and know how to carry a patient without aggravating his injury. He must also be able to perform other emergency care procedures under distant supervision, through his walkie-talkie radio, of the emergency physician on duty.

If we take into account the ambulance design proposed by the National Academy of Sciences, the broad spectrum of medical and surgical emergencies demanding ambulance service, the essential requirement of immediate, efficient, and safe transportation of a casualty from anywhere in the region to the treatment center, the operation of such highly specialized vehicles as "heartmobiles," and the need to keep cost at a minimum, it becomes clear that the ambulance of the future must be a general purpose vehicle. It must be able to transport all kinds of patients and yet be as simple as possible. Special items of equipment should be incorporated into the ambulance only when it has been demonstrated that during the short period of transportation from the site of the injury to the emergency station, lives will be saved or serious complications prevented.

It is highly unlikely, for example, that during the transportation of patients with acute heart attacks telemetry equipment which would transmit the patient's electrocardiogram to the emergency station could have a significant effect on outcome. Most of the deaths from coronary heart attacks occur before the ambulance can reach the patient. Actually, in the Framingham Heart Study,[4] where a "normal" population has been followed for more than twenty years, about one half of the deaths during the first heart attack occurred instantly, or during

4. W. P. Castelli and Patricia McNamara, "Framingham Heart Study," personal communication (July 1973).

the first hour after the onset of the illness. There was a small increment of less than 8 percent of deaths occurring between the first and eighth hours when most of the transportation would be taking place. During transportation, with a pulse rate monitor functioning, if the patient's life were threatened by an irregular rhythm, a defibrillator or a dose of a drug such as lidocaine in the hands of a well-trained emergency aide should suffice, and little would be added by electrocardiographic biotelemetry.

It is also clear that the use of specialized vehicles for particular purposes in a large regional area would add much inflexibility to the system. It would be impracticable to try to match the specific emergency needs of the patient with the relatively few vehicles that were designed for his particular care. Long delays in transportation to a treatment center would inevitably result. The military experience suggests that it would be more reasonable to have a fleet of general purpose ambulances equipped to handle life-threatening emergencies, operating in a system where the time interval from injury to treatment is kept as short as possible, and where the forewarned treatment center is fully prepared to handle the specific emergency. These conclusions on ambulance design, although obvious at this time, must be tested by actual experiments in the field.

Helicopters have limited but essential functions in an emergency system. Their usefulness is greatest in remote areas where highways are lacking and the distances are extremely great. The helicopter must be able to operate in all kinds of weather and be large enough to transport a patient sheltered from the elements in a horizontal position. Most military helicopters do, and most police and highway helicopters do not, meet these requirements. Moreover, if the time saved is to justify its use, the helicopter pad must be reasonably close to the emergency treatment center. Since the need for helicopter transportation is relatively infrequent and its initial and operating costs are very high, it would be best to arrange for such transportation by agreement, whenever possible, with the nearest military base.

It is unlikely that a few helicopters will solve the difficult problem of transportation of all very ill patients into and out of urban areas during rush hours. Indeed, it would appear that the only choice we will have in the long run is to do away with the private vehicles that create the rush hour traffic. We are trapped by a combination of major crises: the growing energy crisis with limited fuel for private vehicles, the escalating transportation crisis in which the crush of private vehicles is preventing adequate bus transportation,[5] and the worrisome environmental crisis with air pollution from automobile exhausts reaching toxic limits in some areas. These crises interfere with the rapid transportation of patients who need life-saving medical care during rush hours. Whether we like it or not, eventually most personal transportation into and out of cities will have to be provided by highly efficient common carriers combined with intraurban street vehicular transportation.

5. London Transport Executive, *Annual Report and Accounts for 1972* (London, England): pp. 17–18.

Since these crises are already upon us and we cannot arbitrarily cut off personal transportation without a substitute, we must institute effective mass urban transportation at the earliest possible moment.

This trend, by itself, will change the pattern of medical care delivery. After private transportation into the cities is restricted, residential housing in the heart of the cities will be in great demand. In parts of the world where intraurban living has had a high priority, for example, Paris, France, the slums tend to be in a ring just outside the boundaries of the city. This trend has already begun in Boston, Massachusetts. The intraurban slums will disappear as the poor are displaced to the nearby suburbs and medical care delivery will have to be modified to meet this change.

Special emergency vehicles will not be needed for minor emergency cases. Those with minor illnesses or injury who can easily be moved and who need no immediate life-saving care could receive first aid by a specially trained emergency aide in the district reception center (p. 130) or treatment when necessary by a physician in an emergency treatment center in a hospital. In both cases, transportation by taxi, private vehicle, or at times by common carrier when it goes directly to an appropriate emergency station should be adequate. The taxi service could be supplied on a contractual basis with the owners, provided that the drivers received minimal first-aid training and were instructed on the kinds of information that should be transmitted to the command center over the taxi radio. If the emergency service is to be efficient, the general public must know how to call the command center and must follow instructions in regard to the immediate precautions that must be observed and the procedures that must be carried out. They must also know the location of the emergency treatment centers. In an emergency, the triage nurse would give simple advice on the management of the patient and inform the driver of the location of the emergency station to which the patient was to be transported.

The size and distribution of the population served should determine the number of emergency treatment centers. They should be as few as possible and should be deployed among the existing hospitals in a geographic pattern consistent with the incidence of emergency injuries and illnesses. At this first stage of the medical care blueprint, they should, insofar as possible, be congruent with the plans for the evolution of an ambulatory care program in a total regional medical system. Thus, there need not be an emergency treatment center in every hospital. Indeed, because of the requirement of twenty-four-hour coverage, emergency stations can be located only in hospitals having a resident staff or a special team of emergency care physicians. But every hospital must be tied in to the emergency medical service if only to guide to proper care all of the emergency cases coming to its attention. Depending upon hospital resources, availability of specialized physicians and other personnel, laboratory facilities, and equipment, some stations may treat all emergencies, others may treat only medical or surgical cases, while still others may have the professional and technological personnel to provide such highly specialized care as that demanded by cardiac emergencies or head injuries. Eventually, the pattern of emergency care stations in hospitals in a particular area will be integrated into the structure of the regional medical care system.

A well-functioning emergency medical service would meet the needs of physicians and the public. All would learn of the benefits of a systematic attack on an important medical care problem. Since most physicians are not interested in providing twenty-four-hour-a-day emergency service for which they are poorly compensated, they would appreciate the opportunity to refer their emergency cases if they had the assurance that their patients would be well treated. The physician would also become convinced that the introduction of a system per se need not threaten his independence nor the physician-patient relationship. The public would be reassured that their emergency needs would be systematically cared for with immediate access to necessary personnel, equipment, and other resources.

We can no longer be satisfied with the hodgepodge of emergency treatment centers that willy-nilly provide or refuse care to those who knock at their doors. We cannot continue to refer patients "to the nearest hospital" as is provided by police or fire regulations in some of our larger cities, without regard to the nature of the emergency or to the resources available for treatment. Moreover, our limited health budgets cannot tolerate the wasteful duplication of emergency stations in our haphazard lack of system. When we face up to all of these facts, we realize that there is no choice but to create a central emergency authority in each future medical care region to plan, introduce, integrate, test, and supervise all aspects of the system to the end that each emergency patient receives at the earliest possible moment exactly the treatment that he needs.

Ambulatory Medical Care: The Unfilled Gap

6

If anyone is sick enough to need a doctor, but not so ill as to be flat in bed in a hospital, the chances are he will not get the full benefits of modern medical care. In the United States, ambulatory medicine—the care of the patient "on the hoof"—tends to be catch-as-catch-can: particularly, as we have seen, if he has an acute medical or surgical emergency, needs preventive services, is suffering from a minor illness, or is in the early stages of a serious disease. In sharp contrast, in the inpatient services in many of our hospitals, particularly those affiliated with medical schools, the care of the patient may be the best in the world.

In a word, ambulatory care is the great unfilled gap in current medical practice. The implications are serious indeed because it is clear that many of the resources of modern medicine are now not being applied to the prevention of disease or to the treatment of the early stages of serious illness when most can be done for the patient.

The disorganized state of ambulatory medical care makes it difficult for the patient to obtain exactly the services that he needs. This uncertainty increases the total cost of medical care. Delays in diagnosis and treatment, in addition to being harmful to the patient, make the case more costly to treat. The patient with an unsolved medical problem, needing diagnostic study and confused by the disordered state of ambulatory care, seeks out the quiet refuge of the better organized but much more expensive inpatient service of the hospital. Indeed, he eagerly makes this choice when he learns that his insurance policy is more likely to pay for his diagnostic workup if he is treated in the horizontal position in bed rather than in the vertical position as an ambulatory patient.

Since we do not have a single system of medical care for everybody, let us, for guidance in designing the ambulatory care system of the future, examine the pathways that make up our untidy pattern of ambulatory care. Each pathway winds along relatively independent of the others and may or may not conduct the patient along the course best suited to the management of his disease. Access to a particular pathway may depend more on his income, the time of day, his racial background, or geographic location than on his needs for preventive care or for treatment of his illness. The pathways include private care by a physician practicing individually or in a group practice unit, institutional care in the outpatient department or emergency ward of a local hospital, or poverty care in an academic research unit, local community center, or "outreach program."

Private Care

The Private Individual Physician

At the moment, if you are among the fortunate few who have and can afford a personal physician of your own, you can probably reach him or his secretary during the course of the working day. If you can arrange a daytime appointment, you will probably be treated in the doctor's office, often relatively isolated from the complex network of technological facilities and the roster of specialists and allied health personnel that are essential ingredients of modern ambulatory medicine. But if you need your physician when he is off duty, at night, on Wednesday afternoons, on weekends, or when he is ill or on vacation, you will have to deal with the office nurse or the answering service. You may have great difficulty in either tracking him down or discovering which of the physicians covering for him is available to give you immediate care. In the process, you may have to call your friends, a neighborhood nurse, the local hospital, the county medical society, the pharmacist on the corner, or a physician-friend in a distant city.

If you become ill, have no personal physician, and cannot find but could afford one, you may have to figure out for yourself which kind of specialist would be appropriate for the treatment of your condition. Then you will have to try to find one who can care for you promptly. If no emergency exists, you will usually have to wait several weeks for an appointment for ambulatory care, and you may then discover that you picked the wrong kind of specialist. At that point, you may be referred to an appropriate specialist, arrange another appointment, and, after another delay, eventually obtain medical care.

Even at best, most physicians practicing alone can no longer provide modern ambulatory care, which should include immediate access to whatever specialists, allied health personnel, and miracles of modern technology may be needed for the prevention or the treatment of your disease. The isolated doctor's office on the corner of Main and Market Streets is an anachronism that will fade away. These facts lead us to another conclusion. If the individual physician can no longer by himself bring the benefits of modern medical science to his patients, it becomes evident that the constant efforts to attract individual physicians to practice in small rural towns or in the heart of urban ghettos are both shortsighted and misguided. Indeed, they have had a retrogressive effect. The narrow outlook that assumes that the mere availability of an individual practitioner will assure adequate medical care for the patient has resulted in yeomanlike but unsuccessful efforts, using all kinds of inducements, to attract physicians to rural areas. The inability to recruit physicians has led to the enactment of legislation in the states of New York and Massachusetts that certifies a chiropractor to take the place of a physician. If one lives in an area where there are no physicians and no plans for bringing a medical care system to the community, it is understandable that a chiropractor or even a local pharmacist may appear to be better than nothing. But it is a far cry from modern medical care.

Private Physicians in a Group Practice Unit

In order to overcome some of the obvious limitations of individual practice, private group practice units have been developed. They have recently become very popular. Indeed, there has been a flurry of legislative proposals favoring the evolution of group practice units under such euphemisms as "health maintenance organizations." This development is based on the record of the superb ambulatory care and medical consultation provided by the relatively few outstanding group practice centers which consist of a complete roster of specialists, paramedical personnel, and technological resources that are now the hallmark of modern scientific inpatient care. Such group practice units have provided some of the highest quality of ambulatory medical care in our country, particularly when they have been buttressed by prepayment insurance plans. But group practice alone, even when prepaid, is no panacea. As this blueprint unfolds, it will become clear that it is only a link—an essential link to be sure—in a total medical care system.

Two additional words of caution! The term "group practice" has many meanings that may extend from famous well-organized care centers all the way down to an office in which two physicians share the services of a secretary or a small laboratory. Those at the lower end of the range of group practice units do not have the resources to provide modern medical care and must not be included in legislative definitions for future planning.

Instead, in the absence of a national health program, the following definition of a group practice unit established by the Group Health Association would appear to be minimal:

Group medical practice involves the cooperative organization of five or more full-time physicians representing at least three specialized fields of medicine (including internal medicine and general surgery), using common facilities and staff, and sharing responsibility for the provision of comprehensive medical care to a continuing clientele.

But even when such criteria are met, it must be understood that freestanding group practice units separated from the hospital are wasteful of capital investment and of professional and technical personnel. When completely equipped group practice units are separated by distance and time from the hospital and by a lack of close functional interrelationship with it, capital investment in equipment is duplicated, operating costs are high, and physicians' time is wasted in shuttling back and forth between the ambulatory center and the hospital as they try to provide essential care for their ambulatory patients and their inpatients. Group practice is indeed essential. But if a group practice unit is to bring the blessings of scientific and technological medical advance to its patients at a cost that society can afford, it must be complete enough to meet its assigned task and be effectively interrelated with the resources, equipment, and personnel of the inpatient hospital services and of the regional medical care system.

Institutional Ambulatory Care

Ambulatory Care Clinics

If you cannot afford private care and have no personal physician, or if you live in a rural or urban ghetto area where there are no local physicians, it may be extremely difficult, and at times impossible, to find someone to give you ambulatory care. You may report to the outpatient or emergency service of a local hospital if one exists. If not, and you call the local medical society for the name of a physician who might be on duty, his services are not likely to be available without cost. You may actually know that care is available in a distant hospital but cannot reach it because you do not own a car and cannot afford a taxi. Sometimes, because of inadequate finances or geographic inaccessibility, you may simply have to get along without any medical care at all.

During the day, if you cannot afford a private physician, you will be forced to seek ambulatory care in the outpatient department of a hospital if you can get to one. Outpatient departments tend to be run in a relatively mechanical and impersonal fashion, often with interminable delays in unattractive surroundings. Above all, most of them lack the sine qua non of ambulatory care—a personal physician. There is, of course, a wide range of quality in the outpatient facilities of our many hospitals and a few do provide very good ambulatory care. But for the country as a whole, the flat statement can be made that our hospital outpatient departments do not provide modern personal scientific medical care.

At night, ambulatory medical care is even more

inaccessible since outpatient departments are usually closed. Indeed, outside of the working day, private ambulatory medical care may also be almost completely unavailable. For all sick patients, there may be only one resource to turn to at night—the emergency service of the local hospital, if any. The emergency care services of hospitals have become, in effect, twenty-four-hour-a-day outpatient departments, with a smaller and smaller percentage of true emergency cases among the patients coming for treatment. In fact, emergency services in hospitals are often overloaded at night with run-of-the-mill ambulatory patients whose care interferes with the treatment of life-threatening emergencies. For routine cases, emergency rooms in many hospitals are likely to be staffed for relatively short tours of duty by inadequately supervised interns and residents so that ambulatory treatment tends to be episodic with little continuity of care. Physician and patient are usually strangers to each other and unless the physician himself becomes interested in the case, they are unlikely to see each other again.

We may conclude that ambulatory care services in most hospitals do not at the present time provide easily accessible, high-quality, personal, continuing medical care to patients who cannot afford or cannot find a personal physician.

Medical Care Programs for Disadvantaged Populations

The glaring deficiencies in ambulatory medical care in the United States have been sharply focused by recent attempts to extend such care to disadvantaged populations. Although federal financing has been essential and helpful, the nature of medical care in poverty areas has been shaped mostly by local conditions—accessibility to a hospital and to a medical school, availability of empty buildings, the interest and prejudices of physicians, local officials, and residents of the area, and the marshaling of financial resources.

No single national pattern of ambulatory medical care in disadvantaged areas has emerged. The tradition of untidy ambulatory care is preserved and at least three separate kinds of programs have evolved. A few comprehensive units have been established under the direction of medical school faculties or hospital research units, for example, the Columbia Point Program in Boston, and the Martin Luther King Center in the Bronx. They could provide excellent ambulatory medical care, but their cost and elaborate academic professional staffing make them nonreproducible for general application throughout the country. Moreover, those academic experimental medical care units that have been established are having almost insuperable difficulties in recruiting an adequate number of physicians and other professional staff, and some of them are already shut down.

In the second kind of program, representatives of disadvantaged populations and their friends under inspired and devoted leadership, sometimes aided by the local medical school (for example, the Watts Program in Los Angeles), have designed and built treatment centers from scratch. Ambulatory medical care is provided where, for all practical purposes, none previously existed. But such centers tend to be relatively isolated from technological resources and specialists' services and also have great difficulty in physician recruitment. Physicians who do work in local units spend an inordinate amount of time traveling back and forth between their ambulatory patients in the center and their inpatients in the hospital. Indeed, after the initial flurry of excitement and idealism has died down, health departments and other agencies working with local community groups have over the years found it almost impossible to recruit enough competent physicians for long enough periods of time to provide adequate care in centers remote from hospitals. Isolation from professional contacts and hospital resources, inadequate financial compensation, and the waste of professional time in transportation in our heavily trafficked cities or in driving long distances out in the country are probably responsible for the difficulties in recruitment of physicians to practice in ambulatory care units isolated from hospitals.

Finally, ambulatory care has also been provided in disadvantaged areas by the extension, sometimes called "outreach," of existing outpatient hospital services. These efforts have been relatively unsuccessful because of the limitations that are intrinsic to the usual hospital outpatient department. Indeed, the traditional impersonal isolation of the hospital outpatient department tends to be extended out into the community. Except for a few idealistic physicians, the "outreach" program also suffers from great difficulty in physician recruitment.

Double Standard of Medical Care
Above all, the inherent defect in all of the poverty programs is the creation of a double standard of medical care—one for the affluent and the other for the poor.

And yet all these efforts must be applauded, because services are provided in areas where none previously existed. Medical care programs for the poor have certainly satisfied many unmet needs. From a short-range point of view, such efforts have been useful and should be supported. The best must not become the enemy of the good. But we must also take the long view. We must eventually develop a single system of ambulatory services that makes it possible for physicians and paramedical personnel to use all medical care resources efficiently and effectively in a program that fosters personal care and brings all of the benefits of modern scientific medicine to all of our citizens.

Scarcity of General Physicians
This analysis of ambulatory care will not be complete unless we face up to the scarcity of general physicians. The constant increase in complexity of medical care simply demands that one individual—probably a general physician—must be responsible for fitting together the many facets of modern medical care for the benefit of the individual patient. This blueprint assumes the eventual availability of a general physician for everyone. A plan will be proposed for the education of a large number of general physicians to provide ambulatory care. In the meantime, to supply any medical care at all in some areas, compromises will have to be made by substituting medically supervised allied health personnel to perform duties that really demand the services of a physician. Supervision may be immediate and direct or through visual links taking advantage of modern communication,

transportation, and instrumentation technology. But in all such cases, we must be sure through carefully controlled research that no real harm comes to the patient. Indeed, throughout this analysis it is assumed that carefully controlled studies will determine the eventual design of an effective fail-safe ambulatory care system.

How then can we design and test an ambulatory medical care program that will favor a personal physician-patient relationship, implement modern scientific knowledge, incorporate relevant advances in modern technology, supply essential specialist and paramedical services, and apply existing and potential social resources for the benefit of all patients?

The Ambulatory Program of the Future

7

The ambulatory care program of the future will be interrelated with all of the inpatient services of the hospital of the future (figure 1), the emergency care service, and all of the resources of the regional system (figure 2). To effect such interrelationships, the regional command center of the emergency system will have to be expanded and modified to include the triage, communication, and transportation services essential to effective ambulatory medical care. It is assumed in the regional medical care system that each community hospital will provide inpatient service to its total service area and be the focal point of a group of ambulatory care districts each serving a local medical marketing area. The location, size, and number of the districts affiliated with each community hospital will depend upon geography, community loyalties and traditions, and the pattern of existing and contemplated communication and transportation systems and highways. With these interrelationships in mind, let us define the governing principles and the essential ingredients of an ambulatory medical care system, go through the stages of its organization, and demonstrate how the individual would be cared for and benefited.

Where Shall the Patient Be Treated?

Two widely disparate kinds of location must be compared in order to plan for the treatment of the ambulatory patient in the future. In the first, freestanding ambulatory medical care centers with functional relationships to but with geographic separation from the community hospital would be built within each district to provide the patient with immediate access to his physician. In the other, the patient would travel to an ambulatory care center immediately adjacent to the inpatient services of the community hospital, where his physician could take advantage of its technological resources, specialists, and paramedical personnel.

At first glance, the freestanding center would seem to be better. Immediate access for the patient and the location of the center within the community would appear to outweight the separation of the physician from his hospital. Moreover, this pattern maintains the tradition of having your own doctor nearby and would, therefore, be more acceptable. But actual experience in bringing high-quality ambulatory medical care to the patient by this method has uncovered a number of almost insurmountable obstacles. As I have pointed out, it has been literally impossible to recruit an adequate number of physicians who would be willing to practice for any significant period of time in centers geographically isolated from the hospital. The physician, educated in a hospital, has learned to practice his profession with the resources of modern medicine immediately at hand. Furthermore, the isolated location of the center wastes much doctor's time—the scarcest medical resource—as he dashes back and forth between the center and the hospital in striving to give good care to both his ambulatory and his hospitalized patients. In some areas, where physicians are simply not available, care is now provided in local centers by a yet to be validated and probably unsatisfactory method of medical care, that is, by assigning immediate and primary responsibility to a nurse-practitioner or a physician's assistant who, when he deems it necessary, can obtain the advice of a physician over the telephone or can refer the patient to a distant hospital.

Those responsible for the administration of freestanding ambulatory medical centers are torn between trying to meet most of the physician's technological needs in the isolated center, and yet not wasting scarce financial resources by purchasing duplicate expensive items of equipment or by building laboratories to provide services already available in the nearest hospital. Usually, when ambulatory care is given in freestanding centers, the location of the laboratory where the test is performed depends on its complexity. Simple urine, blood-counting, and blood-chemistry tests are easily performed in laboratories in isolated centers. But other frequently useful tests, such as a chest x-ray or an electrocardiogram, requiring complex equipment or special installation and high-level interpretation are much more difficult to arrange. As a result, the more complicated tests are not usually performed at isolated centers. Therefore, the patient must travel to the hospital, and the advantage of convenient geographic location of the isolated ambulatory care center is lost. The situation is particularly onerous when it becomes necessary to perform repeated tests on the same patient. Moreover, under such circumstances, records, reports, and films shuttle irregularly back and forth between the center and the hospital as attempts are made to keep up with the needs of the patient. Finally, the patient will always have to be transported to the hospital for the performance of unusual or complicated tests that are necessary for his diagnosis or management.

Freestanding centers are also limited by the awkwardness, the expense, and at times the impossibility of arranging for certain ambulatory care services required for patient care. Specialists, for example, may not be able to provide service in an isolated center because it lacks unusual items of equipment or specially trained technical assistants. They would also have to waste much valuable professional time in travel. Immediate appointments, even when imperative, may at times be impossible to arrange. Allied medical personnel also have special needs that govern the site where treatment is administered. Some allied medical personnel such as physiotherapists or laboratory technicians need equipment to perform their functions; others may require immediate medical supervision, for example, physicians' assistants performing minor surgery; or they may increase costs by providing duplicating services already available in the nearest community hospital.

Whenever a patient has to go to the hospital for ambulatory care, he loses the advantage of the local geographic accessibility of the ambulatory care center and is thereby forced to get his treatment at two separate sites. Finally, we can be sure that as medical care becomes ever more complicated, it will become more and more impractical for the patient to obtain at the freestanding isolated center all of the services of general physicians, specialists, and allied health personnel and the laboratory and technological resources that constitute excellent continuous ambulatory medical care.

Let us now consider the alternative of locating the ambulatory care center at the hospital. Professional personnel will have the great advantage of immediate access to all of the available medical care resources required for ambulatory care. But now a new difficulty arises. The patient is geographically separated from the treatment center and his personal physician and all ambulatory services become relatively inaccessible to him. The inadequacies of modern mass transportation make the situation worse. In urban areas, common carrier transportation is not available throughout the day and night. Indeed, it is least satisfactory in poverty and ghetto areas where it is most needed for medical care and where taxi transportation may simply be unavailable or cannot be afforded. In rural areas, where there are relatively few physicians, long distances will have to be traveled by the patient to obtain any medical care at all.

Lack of immediate accessibility of ambulatory care may actually be harmful to the patient. Unless an emergency medical care system is established, there may often be serious delays in his treatment when he is critically ill. But even if emergencies are well cared for, patients with early disease if not acutely ill may, because of the awkwardness of the service, tend to postpone their medical care, sometimes with serious results. Perhaps more important, preventive care, which lacks dramatic urgency, may be neglected by a large proportion of the population. Finally, because hospital-based ambulatory care will be a new experience for many patients, it will not become effective until patients learn to change their pattern of obtaining medical care.

So we see that modern efficient ambulatory care cannot be provided entirely either in an isolated center within the patient's geographic area or in a treatment center in a distant community hospital. A more thoroughgoing program is needed.

The Composite Plan

To resolve this dilemma, a composite plan is proposed (figure 3). The proposed program with its special communications and transportation systems will give the patient easy access to his physician whenever he needs him. But when physician's services are not required, he will receive standardized preventive services such as immunizations and screening examinations and treatment for specified minor illnesses—for example, upper respiratory infections or the hives—and simple first aid—for example, cuts not requiring stitches or localized first- and second-degree burns—from appropriately supervised allied medical personnel in the reception center in his district. The proposed plan has the further advantage that the physician in the treatment center adjacent to the inpatient services of the hospital will have easy access to the essential facilities, services, technological resources, and personnel necessary to provide high quality ambulatory medical care. The plan, pending the education of an adequate number of general physicians, also allows for an interim compromise in which moderately ill patients, who really should be cared for by a physician, could be treated by a nurse-practitioner or a physicians' assistant if he were supervised by a physician either directly, or distantly through a television or other visual communications link.

Essential Elements of an Ambulatory Program
The essential elements of an effective ambulatory care program include:
1. a treatment center for medical and dental care adjacent to the hospital (figure 3), where the patient's physician will have his office and have access to specialists, allied health personnel, and technological and rehabilitation resources;
2. a general physician reincarnated in modern dress who as "captain of the team" will be primary physician, personal physician, and pilot physician to his patient;
3. a new system of medical education in which each physician graduate will have completed a course of study specifically designed for his future professional role in the practice of medicine or in research;

4. a district reception, triage, and minor treatment, first-aid, and rehabilitation center convenient to the patient and manned by allied medical personnel;
5. a communications system centered on the emergency command center with subunits in the reception center in each district to guarantee the most effective use of all regional resources in the care of the individual patient;
6. a special transportation system linking the home of the patient, the reception center in the district, the treatment center at the community hospital, and the central regional hospital and other resources of the regional system;
7. a center for temporary care of children when the responsible parent is receiving preventive or therapeutic ambulatory care;
8. a health-alerting system to suspect, identify, and refer to care people who have preventive and therapeutic needs; and
9. an education program for the public so that they can use the system effectively, and for the staff to maintain the service at an optimal level.

The Treatment Center

The treatment center at the community hospital will house the general physician and will be the locus of physicians' services for ambulatory patients. A patient who needs a physician's care will be referred by the triage nurse in the reception center in his district to his personal physician in the treatment center. The center itself must be so attractively designed, its furnishing so warm and welcoming, and its staff so friendly that patients will willingly come to it, not only for the treatment of specific complaints but for preventive services. There is a great danger that the establishment of a system of medical care will by its very nature favor the evolution of impersonal, faceless, and mechanical services—that is, it will exacerbate the unpleasant aspects of the present outpatient department environment. To counteract this tendency, the ambiance of the center must be warm and friendly, clean and quiet, with comfortable waiting spaces, adequate toilet facilities, and convenient parking for all types of vehicles, including baby carriages.

The proposed treatment center might at first glance seem to be inordinately expensive. But further analysis suggests that the building of an inviting ambulatory care center at the hospital would prove to be a good investment. It should improve the health of the population by facilitating preventive care and the early treatment of serious illness which when successful will decrease inpatient admissions. An attractive and effective ambulatory treatment center would also recoup in great measure the money now wasted by the unnecessary use of the very expensive inpatient hospital services for diagnostic purposes, for minor treatment, and for other procedures that do not require immobilization of the patient in the horizontal position. At present, patients are driven by helter-skelter and at times inadequate and often unavailable ambulatory care facilities, and unbalanced insurance programs to seek the warm security of the hospital bed whenever they are threatened by potentially serious illness. If the ambulatory care service were friendly and effective, the patient would be more willing to fit his medical care into his daily life pattern, and the result would be to cut down on costs and permit him to live a more normal existence. Toward this end, the appointment system will have to be flexible enough to gear ambulatory medical care procedures into the employment schedules and family demands of the individual patient.

The treatment center must be strategically placed within the structure of the hospital so that the general physician may conduct his practice in an efficient manner. It should be located peripheral to the complex maze of the inpatient services of the hospital associated in the mind of the layman with serious or fatal illness. Since the treatment center will be mainly concerned with relatively less critical medical problems and with physicians' preventive services for well people, these should be reflected in its location and in its structure.

Although for diagrammatic clarity, the ambulatory care center is shown as a separate unit (figure 1), economies of structure and financing and more efficient function would probably be achieved if the ambulatory care center were located in the same building with the emergency station, the preventive care services, the offices of the specialists and of certain allied health personnel such as physicians' assistants and technicians, and the laboratories performing routine procedures. In any event, there must be effective functional relationships via the internal communication and transportation systems with all laboratory, x-ray, and other technological resources, the roster of specialists, the panoply of allied medical services, the computer facilities, and the record library, and with the inpatient services when hospital admission is required (figure 3). These interrelationships will be helpful in two ways. All available resources will be accessible for the care of the ambulatory patient. Moreover, the general physician will be able to provide continuity of care whenever his patient is admitted as an inpatient or is treated elsewhere in the hospital. Before continuing with the description of the proposed ambulatory care system, it is necessary to examine the role of the general physican within it.

The General Physician: The "Captain of the Team"

8

As the potential of modern medical care constantly increases, its implementation becomes ever more complex. It is no longer feasible for an individual doctor, working alone without specialists, technology, or allied health personnel, to identify, apply, and fit together for each patient the many different components that constitute modern medical care. The components that aid in the maintenance of health and expedite the diagnosis or management of illness include:
1. every relevant item of medical knowledge;
2. the experience, judgment, and skills of all the different kinds of specialists;
3. the services of all needed allied health personnel;
4. preventive, diagnostic, and therapeutic technological developments, including medical instruments (such as for laboratory analysis, and surgery), mechanical devices (such as pacemakers, hearing aids, eyeglasses, and artificial limbs), and medical equipment (such as

x-ray and electrocardiograph), and communication and transportation equipment and facilities;
5. drugs, vaccines, serums, and other preventive and therapeutic agents;
6. the institutional, financial, and social resources required to implement care; and
7. last, but not least, a general physician to perform the essential role of the "captain of the team."

Let us examine the role, responsibilities, and duties of the "captain of the team." As we do, it will become clear that he must be a generalist physician educated specifically for this task. He will be responsible for supervising the total care of his patients, and, with the aid of technology and the assistance of whatever allied health personnel he may need, will himself provide ambulatory care.

Depending upon the needs of his patients, the general physician will provide many different kinds of essential services. For primary care, he will be the first physician to see and evaluate his patient. He will initiate care and call upon any needed resource in the medical care system for more precise diagnosis or for the immediate management of the patient or for both. In so doing, he must practice anticipatory medicine—that is, he will perform preventive procedures such as removing a precancerous skin lesion and will himself identify and treat or arrange for specialist's care in the early stages of serious life-threatening illness such as congenital heart disease. As personal physician, he will supply guidance, reassurance, and support, and become the medical pilot for the patient and his family. As pilot physician, he will bear the serious responsibility for continuity of care, which, in essence, means identifying and fitting together all facets of modern medicine for total ongoing care of, for example, vascular disease causing inadequate circulation to the legs and feet, and for the special requirements of the patient who may also be a diabetic.

How will the general physician care for his patient within the structure of the proposed medical care system? The patient will be referred to his physician in the treatment center of the hospital by the triage nurse at the reception center whenever the patient's medical condition demands a physician's services. After initial evaluation by the physician, appropriate tests will be ordered and when necessary the patient will be referred for specialist consultation and allied medical assistance. The general physician will provide whatever immediate treatment is required and when the patient's workup is completed, he will correlate the results and instruct his patient on the continued management of the illness. This last step may have to be reinforced by allied health personnel in the reception center and by home visits by a public health nurse or other allied health professional person.

When inpatient care becomes necessary, either within the nearby community hospital or in the central hospital of the region, the patient will become the immediate responsibility of the specialist to whom he is referred. All orders for drugs and other treatment relevant to immediate medical care will be written by the specialist. But, such referral does not relieve the patient's general physician from overall responsibility for relating specialists' care to the total management of his patient. To provide continuity of care, the general physician will have to visit his patient on the inpatient services. His visits should give the patient personal reassurance and support. They should also provide opportunities for arranging with the specialist in charge for the required treatment of both the underlying and immediate illnesses. The general physician will also try to anticipate conflicts in patient management and prevent them by forewarning the specialist.

Moreoever, when the general physician actually identifies a contraindicated procedure or treatment, he will alert the specialist either by a note in the patient's record or, when necessary, by seeing to it that the specialist changes the order immediately. Indeed, he will protect his patient in many ways. He must be sure that the treatment of an immediate specialized problem does not conflict with the treatment of any other illnesses of the patient. For example, artificial kidney treatment may remove drugs from the bloodstream that may be essential for treatment of another disease, such as aspirin for arthritis or dilantin for epilepsy. The general physician must ascertain that a drug prescribed for the immediate disease may not have harmful effects on another illness of the patient—for example, belladonna prescribed for the relief of spasm associated with a peptic ulcer may aggravate early glaucoma, a disease that leads to blindness. The patient's physician must also be sure that continued treatment for an underlying disease will not be interrupted during the intensive management of the immediate illness. Thus, whenever an acute illness supervenes, the diabetic patient must continue to receive his insulin, the cardiac sufferer his digitalis and diuretics, and the gouty patient his probenecid—all in proper doses adjusted for the influence of the new illness on the old disease. The patient's physician must also warn the specialist in charge against treatment with a drug to which the patient is known to be sensitive.

The general physician in this proposed system should help to combat the increasing depersonalization of medical care so characteristic of our medical care institutions. An impersonal attitude now pervades the entire hospital, even the best ones. It is clearly heard in the impatient voice of most hospital telephone operators when the call is finally answered. It manifests itself almost viciously at hospital admission as the patient sits and suffers untreated through prolonged interrogation, often on economic matters. Then, with his symptoms still untreated, the patient waits in the admission area for the physician to see him, after which he may become almost frantic at the delays that prevent him from being settled down into his hospital bed. Physicians' care has also tended to become impersonal. For example, in the transfer of a jaundiced patient from the medical to the surgical service of a hospital, continuity of care may now consist of nothing more than the cryptic statement during lunch by the medical to the surgical resident, "We are sending you a gall bladder today." The fact is, that even in our best hospitals nobody is now directly responsible for bringing personal warmth into medical care. Lucky is the patient who has a conscientious personal doctor or comes under the care of a warm, kindly specialist or physician-in-training in the hospital.

The general physician as visualized in this blueprint could stimulate and provide personal care in many ways—by getting patients to accept care, by protecting them against bureaucratic indifference, by helping them to bridge the professional gap, and by providing understanding and reassurance to his patients. Indeed, with the assistance of the resident staff, the general physician would be responsible for introducing warm personal empathy as he supervises the continuity of his patient's care, gives ambulatory care, refers his patient into and among the specialized subsections of inpatient care, and accepts immediate responsibility once again when his patient is discharged back into the community. Throughout this entire process of patient management, the general physician could further personalize care by arranging for home visits by such allied health personnel as public health nurses and medical social workers. The public health nurse would reinforce the physician's instructions by demonstrating their implementation within the household, and the medical social worker would assist in making social resources available to the patient. In a word, the proposed system for the medicine of the future need not be coldly impersonal. Instead, the new general physician as described in this blueprint could provide more personal care than is now available to most patients in our existing nonsystem.

To be sure, without a medical system, if you are fortunate enough to have one of our scarce general physicians, you may already receive many of the services proposed in this blueprint. But in the absence of a system designed to help your general physician at every turn along the way, he wastes much precious time as he performs purely administrative tasks and many other functions that could easily be delegated to allied health personnel or to office staff. Indeed, his present role is so unappealing that medical students do not now seek it out and the chances are that you do not have a general physician. In such circumstances, the more conscientious physician specialists are often forced to allocate a significant proportion of their working day to making sure that all of the different specialists' services interdigitate properly and bring unity into the total care of their patients. Such specialists are deeply grateful whenever they find that a patient has a well-trained general physician to perform this function.

You may now receive some of the individual services of the general physician from one of the growing number of proliferating varieties of allied health personnel. But without a definition of the role of each of the allied health professions, these services tend to be fragmented and chaotic, and if you do not have a general physician, they are often not integrated with your total care. More important, there is remarkably little experimental evidence to document the safe and effective transfer of individual clinical tasks from the general physician to a particular allied health profession. In the proposed system, the role of each allied health profession would be defined, and evidence would be collected concerning the specific clinical tasks of the general physician that could safely and effectively be transferred by him to one of the allied health professions. With such documentation, the general physician could assign many tasks to allied personnel and with the help of modern telemetry and other technology could accept responsibility for the safety and efficacy of their performance and for their appropriateness to your need and their relevance to your total care.

The physician's assistant deserves special mention. Many claims have recently been made that he might actually replace the general physician in medical care in the future. It should be clear from this analysis of the role of the general physician, that the physician's assistant could not conceivably perform as a primary, personal, and pilot physician and act as "captain of the team." But this does not mean that the physician's assistant could not play an essential role in your future care.

The general physician could delegate a large number of important tasks to the physician's assistant, provided that certain criteria are met. We must bring precision and uniformity into the present chaos in the recruitment, education, and the assignment of tasks to the physician's assistant. His role must be precisely defined. His ability to perform certain tasks safely and effectively must be documented. His educational curriculum must have been specifically related to his tasks, duties, and responsibilities. It is fortunate that studies such as those at the University of Wisconsin and at the Naval Medical Research Institute, already cited,[1] on many of these points are actively underway. Many more studies will

1. See page 60.

have to be performed and their research results translated into a system of allied medical care under the supervision of the patient's physician.

In the meantime all kinds of compromises may have to be made. But in so doing, the safety and the health of the patient must not be compromised. In isolated areas such as northern New Hampshire, or in crowded ghettos such as in Washington, D.C., where physician recruitment does not meet the need, physicians' assistants may not only have to provide physicians' services for clearly defined and classified types of minor treatment, but they may also have to care for moderately ill patients. If so, the patient should be protected by supervision of the physician's assistant by a general physician at hand or at a distance via a visual communications link. Preliminary observations on the use of visual links, including television, slow-scan television, and pictures transmitted over telephone lines, are promising. Much careful research must be done to identify the advantages and limitations of these methods of communication on the practice of medicine at a distance. In a word, any procedure or service believed to require the education, training, and experience of a competent physician should not be transferred to a physician's assistant until the safety and efficacy of such practice is documented by careful studies. The converse is also true. When the safety and efficacy of a clinical task performed by a physician's assistant has been established, the physician whenever possible, should delegate that task to him. Eventually, as the criteria of this blueprint are satisfied, a system will evolve defining appropriate roles for the physician and the physician's assistant and all other allied medical personnel as they work together in the care of the patient.

The Trend from General Physician to Specialist

Our plan for the reincarnation of the general physician in modern dress for the medicine of the future will be better understood if we briefly review the history of the decline of the general physician. The shift from general physician to specialist during the past four or five decades was the inevitable result of the rapid flowering of scientific medical advance that demanded increasing specialization for its implementation.[2] The enormous benefits of specialized medical care were soon appreciated. But the mad dash towards specialization obscured the fact that total medical care is more than the sum total of individual specialists' services. It was not really understood that good medical care required the services of both specialized and general physicians. Instead, the general physician was simply forgotten as changes in medical practice and medical education concentrated on the growing role of the specialist in medical care and in research.

The drift towards specialized careers in medicine led to widespread professional and social acceptance and a larger income for the specialist. The specialist received well-deserved professional recognition for his mastery of increasingly difficult scientific theory and for his ability to apply the knowledge in his narrow field in skillful and

2. For a detailed description of the evolution of the specialist and the disappearance of the general practitioner, see D. D. Rutstein, *The Coming Revolution in Medicine* (Cambridge, Massachusetts: MIT Press, 1967): pp. 62–66.

life-saving ways in his workshop in the hospital. Eventually, the establishment of specialty boards placed the formal seal of approval on the superior professional status of the specialist.

In the meantime, as specialist qualifications for hospital appointment were established and upgraded, the general practitioner was downgraded and he was progressively forced out of the hospital. A double pattern of medical care developed with the specialist in the hospital and the general physician in his isolated office in the center of town or, more infrequently, practicing as a member of a medical group located outside of the hospital. Particularly in the more prestigious hospitals, there was no place at all for the general practitioner except when he was invited as an auditor at clinics where his patients' illnesses were under discussion. It is remarkable that even in countries with well-developed systems of medical care, such as the United Kingdom and Sweden, this split pattern persists with the specialist practicing within the hospital and the general physician expected to conduct all of his practice on the outside.

The social status of the specialist grew with his professional reputation. Individuals who could afford to pay his fees, sought him out and took pride in having been treated by a specialist and, by inference, lent their weight over the years to the gradual downgrading of the general physician. Dramatic procedures such as heart surgery or artificial kidney treatment outshone the at least equally important but relatively prosaic preventive and therapeutic management of the individual patient. With the increase in social status for the specialist came greater financial rewards. The public became willing to pay large fees for highly specialized procedures and yet complained bitterly if the general practitioner increased his fee by only a few dollars. Somehow, although there was a constant complaint about not being able to find a doctor, very little was done about it. Rural communities did offer many incentives in their unsuccessful efforts to attract general physicians. But there was no groundswell. In contrast with the numerous societies concerned with the prevention of cruelty to animals, there was not one devoted to the preservation of the general physician.

It did not take long for medical students to recognize the higher professional status of the specialist and the change in public attitude. Most of them opted for specialist careers. With the rare exception of an occasional dedicated student, only those at the bottom of the class who lost out in the intense competition for hospital appointments in special fields drifted off into general practice. Although medical students in recent years have shown greater interest in general practice, it is not likely that many of them will be lured away from specialization until the professional and social status of the general physician and his financial rewards are made commensurate with the importance of his duties and the seriousness of his responsibilities in the total picture of future medical care.

The Rebirth of the General Physician
If we are to enjoy the benefits of the medicine of the future, we must face up to the fact that a large number of general physicians in modern dress will be essential to fit

together the many facets and the increasing complexity of medical procedures and resources for the effective management of the individual patient. The education of a large number of general physicians is the most critical emergency in planning for the medicine of the future. It will also be the most challenging step in this entire blueprint because its accomplishment will require:
1. a decision that general physicians must be educated;
2. a reorientation of all physicians and allied medical practitioners;
3. a dedicated investment of educational resources and personnel;
4. a refocused medical education program;
5. a reshaped and balanced medical curriculum;
6. a change in attitude toward medical care by the average individual in our society; and
7. a willingness to provide adequate financial rewards to those who select this career.

But if the essential role of the general physician in the medical care of the future is recognized and accepted, the task will not be a hopeless one.

In order to recreate the general physician, this proposed blueprint is designed to eliminate many of the undesirable conditions that originally led to his gradual disappearance. In a word, the general physician would no longer have a peripheral, isolated relationship to medical care. Instead, he would have to have a central role in medical care because without his services all of the facets of modern medicine could not be brought to bear efficiently for the benefit of each individual. Moreover, his role will become ever more important as medicine continues to become more fragmented and more complex.

Assuming that the proposed system in this blueprint will assure the patient easy access to care, the general physician's direct responsibility for ambulatory care will demand that his office be in the hospital, where specialist consultation, allied medical services, and technological assistance will be immediately available. His general responsibility for total care will require equal status with the specialist, commensurate financial rewards, and a constant intimacy with the new miracles of medicine as they develop. These growing responsibilities and his improved professional and social status as captain of the team will once again attract medical students to this calling, provided that the medical schools readjust their sights, redefine their objectives, and accept the challenge of educating physicians for the medicine of the future.

The Different Roles of General Physician and Specialist

The future role of the general physician in the proposed plan is so important, so revolutionary, and so different from that of the specialist that this blueprint must contrast his role with that of the internist (specialist in internal medicine) and with specialists in general so that their contributions to medical care and the principles differentiating the education of the general physician from that of the specialist are clearly understood. Just as *the general physician is directly responsible for ambulatory care* and for general overall supervision of the continuity of care of his patient in all stages of health and disease, so will *the internist be immediately responsible for inpatient care* and for episodic and continued consultative supervision of complicated generalized disease, such as chronic anemia, kidney failure, and Hodgkin's Disease.

The clinical responsibilities of the general physician as he supervises the total care of his patient will focus on the prevention of disease and disability, on the precise differentiation between the initial symptoms of a serious illness from those of run-of-the-mill minor illnesses, and on the specific and symptomatic treatment of the diseases that commonly afflict mankind. He must not waste his time on the esoteric details of rare museum-piece illnesses that constantly hypnotize the specialist.

In contrast, the internist will concentrate on difficult diagnostic problems, the treatment of acute severe illness or life-threatening exacerbations of chronic illness. Most internists will become qualified in one of many narrow subspecialties of medicine, such as cardiology or gastroenterology, or kidney, chest, or blood disease. In his subspecialty, the internist will have intimate and up-to-date knowledge of the theoretical mechanisms of certain illnesses reinforced by extensive experience in the practical management of many patients seriously ill with these same diseases. Most important, his more narrowly focused interest should make it possible for him to be aware of the many ramifications of each illness and be able to separate its natural history from its modification by drugs and other therapeutic agents.

In a word, the general physician will be the patient's own doctor and as captain of the team will be responsible for total preventive and therapeutic anticipatory medical care, while the internist will consult episodically or at times maintain continuous consultative supervision whenever intensive, theoretical, and practical knowledge of and experience with the disease in question are essential for the optimal care of the patient. Thus, the general physician will observe his patient with a wide-angle lens, while the internist will focus down with his magnifying glass. Moreover, all other clinical specialists will share the care of the patient with the general physician in the same way.

In the ambulatory medical care program of the future, let us now leave the treatment center and the duties and responsibilities of general physicians within it and, turning to the role of the reception center in the "health district," follow the channel that the patient would take in obtaining ambulatory care (figure 3).

The Reception Center   9

The reception center conveniently placed in the heart of the local medical service area, that is, in one of the districts affiliated with each community hospital, will be the focal point of contact between the public served, the staff of the ambulatory care system, and all other medical facilities in the district. It will be the location of many important services, among them:
1. medical care guidance, so that everyone may be referred to the kind of preventive or therapeutic care that he needs when he needs it, including the preventive and therapeutic services of his physician;
2. continued reassurance to patients with clearly diagnosed minor illnesses who have unfounded worries that they are seriously ill;
3. well-baby care;
4. medical care not requiring the services of a physician, including first aid for minor emergencies;
5. home visiting services;

6. health alerting functions and health education;
7. school health services;
8. the communications and transportation subcenter of the regional system; and
9. a meeting place for medical care staff and for committees of consumers for program evaluation and improvement.

As an interim compromise, if the number of general physicians is inadequate, provision may also have to be made in some districts to permit allied medical personnel to manage moderately ill patients under the direct or distant guidance and supervision of the physician by means of a television or other visual link between the reception center in the district and the treatment center at the hospital.

Patient Referral System in Ambulatory Care

The crucial service of the reception center is reliable referral of the patient to exactly the medical care that he needs. This system in the reception center will reproduce in miniature the triage system in the regional command center governing the entire ambulatory and emergency medical care program. As in the regional command center, triage will be performed by a nurse with the assistance of a physician by telephone as needed. She will refer residents of the district to the patient's physician in the treatment center at the hospital for therapeutic or preventive care; to the nurses or other allied health personnel in the district reception center or in the treatment center at the hospital for treatment of minor medical care problems specifically allocated to them; to the emergency medical care system; to a particular allied health profession for home health care; or, under special circumstances after consultation with the patient's physician, directly to a particular specialist in the community hospital or in the central hospital in the regional system.

No medical care system can be successful unless every sick patient really needing a physician's care is seen by his own doctor at the earliest moment. Indeed, the channel to the patient's physician in the treatment center adjacent to the hospital must be so effective that his life and health will be fully protected. He will also quickly discover that the new ambulatory system works better than the present "catch-as-catch-can" method of arranging an appointment with a doctor. It will no longer be necessary for the very sick patient to struggle with the telephone book and the physician's secretary to locate his physician or his physician's associate who covers for him on nights, weekends, and holidays. In the proposed ambulatory care system, the communications post in the reception center will become a subunit of the communications command center of the entire regional system. The communications system must operate so that the patient will simply call the single telephone number of the medical care system, and all of the activity will go on behind rather than in front of the switchboard. When the patient needs the services of his own doctor, a simple computer program will guide the triage nurse and the telephone operator in reaching him or the colleague covering for him. We do not have to wait for the creation of a national health program to set up an efficient communications system of this sort between doctor and patient. It would be an immediate boon for both the patient and the practicing physician.

If the sick ambulatory patient is to receive effective medical care from his physician, a convenient appointment with his doctor will not be enough. The appointment must be fixed at the place where the patient may be treated most effectively, in most instances at the treatment center adjoining the community hospital. The triage nurse will arrange all the preliminary details, including routine laboratory tests essential to an effective and satisfactory visit to the physician. When time permits, and only upon order of the physician, she will arrange for specialist's consultation or scheduled special laboratory and other tests, including measurements to be made by allied medical personnel, such as audiometry or muscle testing. The triage nurse will activate the information-processing system so that the test results will be included in the patient's record, which must be immediately at hand or retrieved by a computer before the physician sees the patient. The nurse will also arrange for the patient to be at the treatment center at the appointed time. The communication and transportation systems must be designed to facilitate all of these steps in ambulatory care. The triage nurse in the reception center will be responsible for all of these and any other arrangements necessary for a successful visit of the patient with his physician.

A word of caution. The triage nurse, working in the triage system, or a physician's assistant in the reception center will *not* serve as a first-line physician for the patient. Medical triage is concerned with the decisions as to whether, when, and where a physician's services are needed. It is not a procedure whereby someone other than the physician acting alone makes a preliminary medical diagnosis on the patient. If the patient is ill enough to need a diagnosis, he should be guided to a physician who has available to him all the background, knowledge, and experience, the technological resources, allied health personnel, and specialists needed to perform that complicated task.

The difficulty of ascertaining the history of a patient's present illness illustrates how impossible it is at this point in time to delegate the primary evaluation of a patient's illness to a physician's assistant working alone without medical supervision.

A complete, reliable, and relevant history of the patient's present illness is the key to precise diagnosis and to his immediate care. Of all of the tasks performed by the physician, none makes more demands on his knowledge, background, education, training, and experience than gleaning the facts of the present illness from the patient and fitting them into a diagnosis, or a set of diagnostic patterns. This process is much more difficult than the random procedure of eliciting past medical, family, social, or occupational history which can be collected relatively easily through varying combinations of questionnaires, self- or physician's assistant- or nurse-administered, and different types of computer programs. Even the ascertainment of simple facts of the present illness, such as its duration, so important to diagnosis, may be complicated. Patients may be poor observers and may have faulty memories. It may be necessary for the physician to ask the same simple question in many different ways to find out exactly what did happen. For example, a patient may be asked on February 1st, "How long have you been sick?"—"About two or three weeks." —"Were you ill on New Year's Day?"—"Yes"—"On Christmas?"—"Yes, I didn't eat much of the dinner."— "On Thanksgiving?"—"I was okay then, it probably started a week or two before Christmas."

Each question asked by the physician on eliciting the facts about the present illness, depends on the patient's answers to previous questions and on the physician's understanding of the ways in which groups of symptoms may fit together in the many diagnoses he is considering as he interrogates his patient. The physician has to be very skillful to elicit an exact description of a symptom whose variations may point to one or another disease. If, for example, the sick patient says he has pain in his right upper abdomen, the physician will obtain a complete description of the pain, including time of onset, duration, exact location, severity, character, recurrence, and the other parts of the body to which the pain is referred. But, he will not stop there. As he goes through the process of synthesizing, comparing, and analyzing patterns of illness, he will also inquire about the other symptoms of the many possible diagnoses that he knows may produce pain in the right upper abdomen. These may be as varied as gall bladder disease, peptic ulcer, pancreatitis, broken rib, pneumonia of the right lower lung, kidney stone, and coronary disease. The physician has to call upon all of his knowledge and ingenuity to find out what really did happen and to synthesize a diagnosis. When this is impossible, he defines a set of patterns—a differential diagnosis—later to be sorted out with the aid of specialists and the laboratory. To be sure, most ambulatory patients have less complicated illness. But the graveyards are full of patients who were treated symptomatically for very early manifestations of serious disease that were ascribed to minor illness. The diagnostic process must be so carefully defined that errors are kept to a minimum.

There is a corollary to this reasoning. Until carefully controlled studies demonstrate otherwise, it is dangerous for the physician to delegate sole responsibility for the primary diagnosis of a patient to a computerized medical device, to a nurse, or to a physician's assistant. The computer can be very useful in assisting the physician to make a diagnosis, but it has not yet been validated as a safe method for the evaluation of the patient's present illness and the establishment of a provisional medical diagnosis.

Similarly, the day may come when it will be demonstrated that a physician's assistant or a nurse can be relied upon to diagnose specific kinds of disease. But before such serious responsibility is allocated to allied medical personnel, prospective controlled studies are needed to document that a specially trained physician's assistant or nurse will make the same range of validated diagnoses as a competent physician. But the qualifications, the role, and the relevant education of the physician's assistant are yet to be defined. At the moment, his assigned tasks, his relatively short period of training, and the content of his curriculum depend on the best guess of whatever person is responsible for any one of the many different training programs now being conducted throughout the country. And, the effectiveness of a nurse in diagnosis is also yet to be validated. Until their reliable performance in diagnosis is documented, the patient requiring precise diagnosis must be cared for by a physician.

But it is not enough to say that the patient must be cared for by a physician. The physician himself makes many errors in diagnosis. Computer programs can be written to provide a fail-safe mechanism for the physician in differential diagnosis and to check on his diagnoses so that errors can be kept to a minimum. The computer can print out a list of all possible diagnoses that should be considered by the physician as he diagnoses a complicated case having a specific set of symptoms, physical findings, and abnormal laboratory test results. The computer may also be extremely helpful to the physician in arriving at a diagnosis when most of the needed information can be quantified. There are disturbances of the body—for example, when the acid base balance is upset or when the excretion of urine by the kidneys is impaired. Under such conditions the concentration of many of the substances dissolved in the blood are changed from normal in characteristic diagnostic patterns that are easily and quickly recognized by the computer. There are also diseases of the blood—leukemia, for example—that are diagnosed by direct observation of the blood cells through the microscope. Automated computerized devices are now being developed that will recognize the presence and unusual distribution of abnormal white blood cells which add up to a specific diagnosis.

Technology can also be helpful to the physician in focusing down on a diagnosis. In *The Coming Revolution in Medicine* it was demonstrated that screening tests, based on the patient's chief complaint, could rule out many possibilities before the physician began to elicit the facts of the patient's present illness.[1] Thus, a patient with the chief complaint of pain in the chest would be given an immediate chest x-ray examination, the results of which would be available in a few minutes to guide the physician when he takes the history and performs the physical examination. Similarly, the jaundiced patient as he entered the admission office of a hospital would have an automated examination of his blood for the biochemical disturbances produced by liver disease. These screening tests on ill patients are different from the screening programs on apparently well individuals to detect the presence of previously unknown disease which is better treated early than late (see chapter 13). But all of these great advances are still a far cry from "diagnosis by computer."

The inappropriateness at this time of assigning to the physician's assistant the responsibility for primary care of the patient does not mean that he will not be extremely useful in the medical care system of the future. As already demonstrated in chapter 4, "The Medical Manpower Muddle," when the exact roles of medical care personnel are precisely defined, the physician's assistant

1. D. D. Rutstein, *The Coming Revolution in Medicine* (Cambridge, Massachusetts: MIT Press, 1967): pp. 99–107 and 143–145.

will become a key figure in performing essential and at times life-saving tasks that do not require the knowledge, education, background, and experience of the physician. If these steps are accomplished, it will be possible to decrease physician's time per patient and therefore the cost of medical care.

Allied Health Services
When it is clear to the triage nurse in the urban or rural district reception center that the patient's illness falls into a distinct category of minimal illness that does not require the services of the physician, she will arrange an appointment for the patient with the appropriate allied health professional. In accordance with the allocation of defined tasks to specific personnel, and with the local plan for medical care, and depending upon the nature of the treatment and its cost effectiveness, specific allied health care tasks may be performed either at the reception center in the district or at the treatment center in the community hospital. The triage nurse will, as she does for an appointment with the physician, arrange all of the details required to insure complete and satisfactory allied health service, including the scheduling of the appointment, the ordering and reporting of the laboratory findings, the availability of the patient's record, and the transportation arrangements. The findings of the manpower studies allocating specific tasks to the physician and to each category of allied medical personnel would be classified in an up-to-date publication to aid triage and to identify the medical care procedures to be provided by each category of professional personnel.

Preventive Services

Using the same resources and facilities, the triage team will arrange for preventive medical care for all residents of the district. Included would be such preventive services as prenatal, postnatal, infant, and dental examinations, checkups on individuals predisposed to serious illness, and screening tests on members of general and special population groups for the earliest stages of illnesses that are better treated early than late. The preventive services provided by allied health personnel in the reception center in the district will have to be carefully interrelated with those provided by the general physician in the treatment center in the community hospital. Well-baby care is an excellent example. Most of the visits will be made in the reception center where the procedures will be performed by a pediatric assistant. But at stated times in infancy, the baby will need to be seen by his physician for total reevaluation of growth and development and for ruling out underlying congenital disease.

Since the individual person is not stimulated by warning symptoms to seek preventive care, computerized tickler files will be needed to identify for the triage team in the district and for the general physician in the community hospital the time and nature of preventive measures for all the residents of the district so that they may receive their preventive services promptly. The triage nurse will then get in touch with the person in question and make all the arrangements for the preventive service.

School Health Services

This crucial preventive service for children has always been handicapped by its isolation from the practice of clinical medicine. The school health service could be an ideal method of finding remediable defects in children; but if appropriate remedies are to be applied, it must be directly integrated with medical care. In this proposed plan, the school health service would be a part of the total system of medical care. Moreover, there would be financial savings, since there would be no need to set up a completely separate school health service with the traditional administrative and overhead costs. The preschool examination would be performed by the child's own physician. In the school, the individual teachers working with nurses from the district reception center would conduct a continuous program to identify children who require immunization or other preventive services, appear to be below par, have many absences due to illness, suddenly cannot keep up with their class, or develop specific symptoms.[2] Such children would be referred through the triage nurse in the district center to appropriate care. The inclusion of the school health service in the total health care system is an excellent example of how the district reception center would function in providing continuity of medical care for each person.

First Aid and Minor Care

First aid and minor care not requiring the services of the physician would be provided in the reception center by a

2. D. B. Nyswander, *Solving School Health Problems. The Astoria Demonstration Study* (New York: The Commonwealth Fund, 1942).

physician's assistant or a public health nurse, or during a home visit by appropriate allied health personnel. The district service would be geared to the areawide emergency medical care system and the ambulatory treatment center so that any of the resources coordinated by the central emergency care command center would be made available when specifically needed for the care of an individual patient.

Home Visiting Services
The reception center will be the guidance point of all of the home visiting allied health services of the district. There are many examples that demonstrate how home health services could be helpful to people needing care. The public health nurse, supervised from the reception center, could act as an emissary of the physician or perform home nursing services. The nurse-midwife housed in the district center could help prepare the home of a prospective mother for the arrival of a new baby. The public health nurse could assist the homemaker in preparing for the discharge of a chronically ill patient from the hospital. In the case of these more specialized services, it is not now clear whether they could operate more efficiently and at lower cost if allied health personnel were housed in the reception center in the district or in the treatment center of the community hospital. Geographic and other local considerations may be crucial in these decisions. In any event, the home allied health services will be guided from the reception center but studies will be needed for each home health service to determine whether it can best be housed in the

reception center in the district or in the treatment center at the community hospital. Initially, it may be assumed that the more generalized services would be housed in the reception center. The more specialized services might well be housed in the treatment center of the hospital, where the allied medical person could have her skills constantly upgraded by providing services both in and out of the hospital, and where she would have more adequate professional supervision.

Next to efficient physicians' services for the patient, home visiting service by allied medical personnel provides the most important link between the medical care system and the community. This link could be strengthened if, at the very beginning of the proposed ambulatory care program, the home visiting service were coupled with the health alerting system (pp. 232–235). That system should be of great assistance in identifying individuals in the district population who need immediate help or should be carefully followed because they will need preventive care or may be in the early stages of severe illness, have chronic disease, or have been lost to the medical care program.

Communication and Transportation Systems 10

Throughout this blueprint, and particularly in the sections on regional, emergency, and ambulatory care, communication and transportation technology have been interwoven to meet operational requirements and to satisfy the administrative, professional, technical, and consumer needs of the proposed medical care system. The spectrum of technical applications is wide and includes such varied problems as command control centers for emergency and ambulatory care, consultation at a distance, remote supervision of allied health personnel, transportation of critically ill, chronically sick, and well individuals, continuous integration of all relevant information for each patient into a medical record that can be retrieved on demand whenever and wherever the patient is treated, walkie-talkie communications between emergency vehicles and treatment centers, and the scheduling of appointments to bring together the patient, his up-to-the-minute hospital record, and his general physician, appropriate specialists, and allied health personnel at the appointed time and place.

Most important of all, the geographic separation of the physician from his patient will demand that the communications network and the special purpose transportation system provide easy, on-time access of the patient to his physician and to all other medical care services. We all yearn for the days of the home visit by the oldfashioned family doctor. Undoubtedly, there were great advantages to the patient's being treated in his home environment at any hour of the day or night. It might be good if that kind of personal care could be reestablished. But the continuing extension of medical care to all segments of the population, the relative scarcity of professional time, and the medical specialists and the technology they require to perform many essential procedures of modern medical care—all these elements now make home visiting almost impossible. We must, therefore, compensate for this lack with an effective communication and transportation system specially designed to bring the patient, whenever necessary, from his home to his physician at the earliest possible moment. Indeed, a special transportation system for medical care is as necessary as the one we now have for airports.

It is reassuring that existing communication and transportation technology is adequate to get the proposed program under way. But provision must also be made to replace outmoded technology with new developments as they evolve. Moreover, under the pressure of specific problems, new technology must be developed from existing scientific knowledge. An example is the performance of tests requiring very expensive equipment. Lung function studies will probably be developed so that the tests are performed on the patient in bed in the community hospital by elaborate and expensive equipment strategically located at the central hospital.

Implicit in any blueprint for the medicine of the future is the education and the availability of the number and kinds of engineers needed to design, construct, improve, and maintain communications centers and networks, transportation systems and vehicles, and their instrumentation. Both theoretical and practical engineering competence will be needed. Since the communications network and transportation system will tie together and flow into every hospital, engineering competence at all levels must permeate the operation of the hospital itself. The day is long gone when the hospital engineer was limited to tending the boiler and repairing leaking pipes. Furthermore, technicians supervised by the engineer will have been trained to standardize, calibrate, maintain, and repair the medical and scientific instruments and the communication devices upon which the operation of the entire system, and the medical care in each hospital will depend. As an example, the hospital engineering service would, after careful and precise study of alternatives, advise on the purchase of analytical laboratory equipment. Throughout the life of the equipment the engineering service would maintain proper standardization, do preventive maintenance, and keep it in repair. In a word, the physician would be assured that the instruments in his hospital could be depended upon to give him accurate numbers on his laboratory reports. Our academic and technical engineering education institutions must respond to all of these needs and reflect them in their educational programs if day-by-day high-quality medical care is to be implemented in an efficient manner.

Many American communities are in the early stages of planning for communication and transportation systems in medical care. At the moment, the focus is on emergency care, but the method of approach is so haphazard that it will serve as a good guide of what not to do. Much of the difficulty results because so many disparate community groups are involved, including hospitals, police, and fire departments, ambulance companies, the health professions, and the public, and because they fail to understand the need for a totally integrated system. The obvious deficiencies are lack of planning for and implementation of a total emergency medical care system, failure of meticulous integration of medical engineering requirements and decision making without adequate or controlled data. What is needed is a provisional plan for total emergency care in each medical care region—similar to the one proposed in this blueprint—which would be accepted by all of the relevant community groups and be tested by a series of carefully designed and controlled field trials, with continuous modification of the total plan as data are accumulated.

One question is whether medical care in remote areas should be provided by personnel in elaborately equipped vehicles or by the efficient transportation of those needing more than minimal care to the appropriate hospital (central hospital, community hospital, or its affiliated cottage hospital) in the regional system. My guess is that the latter is the better solution, but the final answer must surely depend on the results of controlled field trials. This example has been presented in detail because it is typical of many of the questions that will have to be studied and the answers made clear to every community in the country for the effective application of communication and transportation technology during the entire course of the evolution of a national health program.

The major practical obstacle to the implementation and later to the maintenance of effective communication and transportation in the medical care system will be the increase in cost in both money and personnel. Additional new capital investment and operating expenses will have to be budgeted and more and new kinds of personnel will have to be employed. But much of the increased expenditure should be recoverable from the elimination of waste in our present lack of system. In practice, increments in cost should be balanced against the sum of potential savings. Professional time will be conserved by doing away with unnecessary travel. Redundant laboratory facilities, and the excess of open heart surgical, radiation therapy, neurosurgical, and other superspecialist installations and services will be eliminated. The biggest saving of all will result from the sharp decrease in the required number of hospital beds by transfer of the large majority of patients with diagnostic and simple therapeutic problems from expensive inpatient facilities to the proposed relatively inexpensive ambulatory care service within the same hospital. We must look to our economists to study, analyze, and predict the trends in costs and savings implicit in the establishment of an integrated health program; and to our accountants to provide the economists with the quantitative information upon which their estimates will be based.

A final caution. We will not develop effective communication and transportation systems if physicians and engineers continue to go their separate ways. Meticulous integrated medical and engineering planning is essential if communication and transportation systems are to satisfy the medical care needs of patients in the future.

A complete ambulatory care program and its communication and transportation facilities could replace our existing catch-as-catch-can lack of system and do away with many of its inefficiencies and excessive costs. In order to implement this ambulatory care program, we now turn to the changes that will be required in American medical education to graduate the general physicians, dentists, specialists, research workers, and teachers essential to the operation of the ambulatory program and the total medical care system.

Medical Education for the Future

11

The Changing Pattern of Medical Education
Let us briefly review the changing pattern of medical education as a guide to a plan for the future and for the understanding of the role of the future general physician. During the Flexner era, beginning in 1910, concomitant with the flowering of medical science, there evolved an increasingly specialty-oriented medical curriculum buttressed by an ever-expanding and ever more sophisticated scientific college education. It was fitting and proper that medicine should build and grow upon the best documented scientific knowledge of the time. And that principle remains fundamental to all medical education to this day and for the future.

At midcentury, as the Flexner era began to wane, it became evident that the treasure chest of medical science was becoming so full that it could no longer be entirely included within the student's college and medical school curriculum. Even though there could be no compromise with the principle that medicine must stand on a solid scientific base, it became increasingly obvious that no longer could every individual physician be a master of all scientific medical knowledge. Instead, the curriculum would have to be selective and more clearly focused for each of the many kinds of physicians—general physicians, specialists, research workers, and teachers—all of whose services will be essential in the future.

Pursuant to these happenings, in 1960, when I was concerned about the disappearance of the general physician, I proposed that medical schools provide two medical curricula, one for specialists and the other for general physicians.[1] During the 1960s I expanded this simple and somewhat naive double curricular plan into a multichannel medical curriculum to educate the many different kinds of physicians (including the general physician), needed to conduct research and to provide all aspects of medical care for the patient.[2]

In the meantime, in the mid-1960s there was a sudden realization in many medical schools that the Flexner classic single medical curriculum supplemented by elective courses would no longer suffice. The immediate, almost reflex, response was a sudden shift toward a small core curriculum comprising the knowledge "all medical students must have" and an almost completely elective program to be selected by the student with the aid of a faculty advisor.

1. D. D. Rutstein, "Do You Really Want a Family Doctor?" *Harper's Magazine* 22 (October, 1960): pp. 144–150.
2. D. D. Rutstein, *The Coming Revolution in Medicine* (Cambridge, Massachusetts: MIT Press, 1967): pp. 149–157.

The new curriculum plan at the Harvard Medical School did eliminate the fixed, rigid, single medical curriculum, but it did not specifically meet the need. The pendulum had swung too far the other way. The new curriculum was amorphous and had two major defects. Almost unanimous faculty agreement was required for the definition of the core curriculum with the result that its content consisted of nothing but established orthodoxy. Indeed, the core curriculum actually stifled the student's opportunity to learn about the existence of newer areas in medical science and technology. To gain new perspectives, the student had to have the omniscience to select the proper elective courses. But the student could not intelligently select elective courses when he lacked objective prior knowledge of the potential contribution of such new fields as bioengineering and biomathematics, or the neglected fields of preventive and social medicine, and epidemiology. In effect, to seek out the newer or less orthodox areas of medicine, the student had to play a game of blindman's buff.

The student's task was made even more difficult by the failure of medical faculties to provide the guidance implicit in an integrated curriculum. The medical faculty had abandoned its prime responsibility for assembling the available courses into some logical sequence (as is done by individual departments for the college curriculum) which might, with appropriate elective variation, provide a well-rounded experience for each medical student. Instead, in the new curriculum in medical schools, the student was exposed to the core curriculum and was given a faculty advisor and a thick book of elective courses from which he was expected to select the rest of his curriculum. The latter proved to be a large uncharted wasteland containing many scattered and disconnected oases of medical disciplines and knowledge. Furthermore, faculty advisors working in highly specialized fields could not possibly know enough about all of the elective courses to make up for the failure of the total medical faculty to perform its basic task. With whatever help he could obtain from his advisor, the medical student had to substitute his lack of experience for the faculty's failure to act and then formulate his own medical curriculum mostly along the lines of the old Flexner curriculum and by hearsay. As a result, the medical school education of many individual students was misshapen and unbalanced. Fortunately, the defects of the new core plus elective course curriculum have been rapidly recognized, and its era is already coming to an end.

A Multichannel Curriculum: The Only Solution

It has become increasingly clear that the educational needs of the future medical student can be served only by a multichannel medical curriculum designed to educate him for a specific career. The design and implementation of such a curriculum will challenge medical faculties and their deans because it will force them to expand their horizons. They will have no choice but to relate medical education not only to the growth of basic knowledge, their prime responsibility, but also to social needs, influences, and resources that will affect medical practice and medical research.

The history of the college curriculum provides a sound precedent for the future evolution of the medical curriculum. Educational institutions such as Harvard College, beginning in the early nineteenth century, changed their single curriculum for all students to a completely elective curriculum, and finally to a series of curricular pathways now represented by individual course sequences offered by individual departments and balanced by a distribution of courses in other disciplines. If we take advantage of the historical lessons of the evolution of the college curriculum, it will save us much time, grief, and effort in the development of a realistic medical curriculum directly relevant to future needs in basic and clinical medical research and in medical practice.

Criteria for the Medical Curriculum
The proposed medical curriculum must meet the following set of criteria if the wide variety of doctors of medicine—general physicians, specialists, research workers, and educators—needed for the medicine of the future are all to receive an adequate education.
A. The total curriculum would consist of a series of separate pathways, each concerned with education for a particular medical professional role, plus a neutral channel for the as yet undecided student.
B. Transfer from the neutral to a specific pathway would occur as early as possible. A shift from one specific pathway to another would be permitted to students who wished to change their career objectives and who could, with additional courses, qualify for the new pathway.

C. The curriculum in each pathway, including its elective choices, would be uninterrupted from college admission to the end of hospital training with the university responsible for the entire sweep.
D. There would have to be more than one basic course in each discipline to meet the different needs of the wide spectrum of professional careers.
E. The principles of course concentration in the chosen field and distribution among other fields of knowledge would be followed in order to graduate physicians who are both professionally competent and well educated.
F. The total duration of the medical curriculum would no longer be arbitrarily fixed but would vary depending upon the educational requirements of each professional medical career.
G. Qualifications for admission to medical education would be based on excellence and actual requirements would depend upon the career objective of the applicant.
H. Requirements for the granting of university degrees would vary in accordance with the curricular content of the individual pathways.

A. **The Pathways**

A minimal spectrum of medical educational pathways to accommodate the entire range of future medical careers would include the following:
1. general physician's services;
2. medicine and medical specialties;
3. surgery and surgical specialties;
4. maternal, infant, and child health;

5. neuropsychiatry;
6. dentistry and dental surgery;
7. preventive and social medicine, and administrative medicine;
8. molecular medical biology;
9. bioengineering,[3] biophysics, and biomathematics;
10. a neutral channel similar to the classic Flexner curriculum to be pursued by undecided students up to the point when they make their career choice.

It is assumed that the educational experience of every medical student will include a period of hospital training. Graduates of pathways 1 through 6 will receive the practical experience essential to their clinical careers. Physicians graduating in channel 7 will need a comfortable understanding of clinical medicine for careers in the practice of preventive clinical medicine, clinical epidemiology, or public health specialties such as tropical medicine or medical care delivery, which is nothing more than the practical implementation of clinical medicine within the social and economic framework. Firsthand clinical experience in ambulatory and inpatient hospital care will be essential for effective medical administration of high-quality medical care in the future. Indeed, if channel 7 is meticulously evolved, it would automatically include the essential portions of the present educational program of schools of public health and do away with

3. A bioengineer straddling two different sets of disciplines may eventually perform as an engineer, a physician, or a biologist. This curriculum is concerned only with those who will perform in a clinical role. For a complete discussion of the education of the bioengineer and the various roles in which he may perform, see D. D. Rutstein and Murray Eden, *Engineering and Living Systems: Interfaces and Opportunities* (Cambridge, Massachusetts: MIT Press, 1970): pp. 28–38.

those outmoded institutions. This change would integrate preventive and therapeutic medicine so that a comprehensive attack might be made on major and crucial health problems. Finally, physicians graduating from channels 8 and 9, who plan to perform in a clinical role in medical molecular biology, bioengineering, biophysics, or biomathematics, will need clinical experience and training as has been demonstrated in most medical school M.D.-Ph.D. programs.

B. **Transfer among Pathways**

During the course of their education and as soon as possible after a career choice is made, students would be urged to transfer from the neutral pathway to a more specific one. Medical students who, for good and sufficient reasons change from one career objective to another may shift pathways, just as college students change their fields of concentration if they can satisfy the qualifications for admission to the new channel. Most students who change their career objectives will probably have to spend additional time to satisfy the course requirements of the new pathway at the stage of transfer. It is extremely important for purposes of upward mobility in the national health program that members of the allied health professions who are willing and able to accumulate the additional credits be eligible for consideration for admission to one of the channels of medical education. Promising students who began their college education toward a career other than medicine, if they wish to become physicians and if they are able to make up the course requirements and qualify for admission, should be permitted to transfer to a medical pathway.

C. A Continuous Curriculum

A multichannel medical curriculum cannot be successfully implemented if it is subject to the customary interruptions between college, medical school, and hospital education and training. Instead, in every channel there must be no hiatus in a smooth, integrated curriculum beginning at college matriculation and flowing without interruption up to the time when the student becomes qualified to enter upon his chosen career.

The university would be responsible for a continuous, smoothly integrated set of medical curricula from college admission through medical school and hospital education. The transition between college and medical school would be facilitated by integrating the basic science teaching in both schools and eliminating duplicate departments.[4] If successful, such reorganization should also lighten the financial burden of the university. But to be effective, the premedical science college courses would have to be recast in a medical format and fitted to the educational pathways while yet emphasizing the fundamental value of basic science. This difficult task will require a careful balance between the relatively undifferentiated college approach and the more specific orientation of basic science in the medical schools. Both patterns of basic science education are essential to the future physician and would be welded together to provide a broad comprehension of the scientific method and a clear understanding of the meticulous process of

4. The Carnegie Commission on Higher Education, *Higher Education and the Nation's Health. Policies for Medical and Dental Education. A Special Report and Recommendations* (New York: McGraw-Hill, 1970).

inducing a new principle of medical science. It would be possible in the same way, for example, to integrate college mathematics with medical school teaching in biostatistics and biomathematics. As the social sciences in the college become more quantitative and more objective, their teaching would also be integrated with that of preventive medicine and medical care in the medical curriculum. Above all, in this reorganization of the teaching of the basic sciences, we must focus on the principles and their documentation rather than on the infinite details, so that every physician in the future will have the scientific and the clinical background that will permit him to adjust flexibly to the many changes that will occur in basic science, clinical medicine, and medical care throughout his career.

The continuous curriculum should not be so rigid as to prevent transfer of students from one university to another. Moreover, if the university is to supervise the total sweep of medical education from college matriculation to the end of hospital training, colleges that are independent or are affiliated with universities that have no medical schools will have to establish cooperative programs with universities that do have medical schools. This enhanced flexibility of relationship and increased potential for communication among academic institutions should make it easier for the individual medical school to improve its teaching by reexamining its isolated, inbred, and xenophobic programs and by taking advantage of progress made elsewhere.

We can smooth the transition between medical school and hospital teaching in all of the clinical pathways by the implementation of the regional medical program in this blueprint. The linking of community hospitals in the region with the central hospital affiliated with the medical school could facilitate the education of general physicians and specialists and demonstrate how continuity of medical care depends on close interaction between them. Moreover, participation of the student in the actual provision of high-quality continuous medical care to all of the patients of the region at all stages of illness is the best clinical training for the physician of the future whatever his role. It will also demonstrate to the medical student the essential role of the general physician. In their turn, the students could stimulate useful competition among their region-affiliated medical schools toward the practice of better medicine and to attract better students.

D. **Variation in Basic Courses**

To meet the varying needs of students in different pathways, more than one basic course would have to be offered in each discipline. Each student will have to learn the basic science and clinical knowledge that is necessary for the practice of his chosen professional career. Thus, for example, a student in the maternal, infant, and child health pathway, channel 4, would take an intensive course in obstetrics in which he would learn the underlying basic science principles and the theoretical and clinical aspects of normal and abnormal obstetrics, and would have experience, under supervision, in delivering babies and in caring for prenatal and postnatal patients. But every other student in the medical school, that is, those not in the maternal, infant, and child health pathway, must also become generally aware of the basic science background and clinical pattern of obstetrics and their relevance to the practice of his chosen career. Indeed, every student in every pathway must know how the physician graduates of all the other pathways contribute to care so that he will be able to collaborate more effectively with them for the benefit of the patient. Therefore, a student in, say, the molecular biology pathway would take a different basic course in obstetrics —perhaps one concerned with the interface between that specialty and molecular biology, for example, viral-gene interrelationships during pregnancy, in which he would also be privileged to observe a few obstetrical deliveries and would become aware of the principles of prenatal and postnatal care and the major factors affecting the infant mortality rate. In effect, there would have to be a course for the student concentrating in the pathway, and at least one other course in the same discipline for students in all the other pathways. Thus, for the development of a broad point of view essential to the effective practice of medicine in any field, each student must have taken a concentrated course relevant to his interests and needs in his own field and a more general but relevant course in each of the other clinical specialties.

E. **A Balanced Education**

It is not enough that the medical graduate of any of the pathways be professionally competent in his chosen specialty. Nor is his education complete even if he is also well informed about progress in all other fields of medicine so that he may bring their related benefits to his patients. The physician of the future must be able, in addition, to fit all of medicine constructively into the perspective of the aspirations of man and his hopes for a better society. To make this objective at all possible, medical education must extend beyond science, mathematics, and clinical practice. Following the lead of the educational giants at the turn of this century who brought balance into the college curriculum, the medical student must be made aware of the lessons of history, government, and economics, the growing objective knowledge in the social sciences, and the worlds of literature, the humanities, and the arts. Thus, the concentration of courses in his chosen field would be balanced by distribution of courses across the spectrum of knowledge. Final decisions, therefore, for the curricular content of each pathway cannot be left entirely to the specialists in the field. Broad universitywide policy decisions must establish the constraints within which the curricular content of each pathway will offer an opportunity to each student to become both a competent physician and an educated man.

F. The Total Length of the Curriculum

Under the influence of burgeoning scientific knowledge and increasing specialization, there had been a constant tendency to lengthen the time required to educate a physician. This trend reached a peak several decades ago with four years of college, four years of medical school, and, depending upon the specialty selected, three to seven years of hospital training and/or laboratory experience. Then, under the increasing pressure to graduate more physicians, the situation began to reverse itself. Some medical schools arbitrarily shortened the period of college and medical school education required for the M.D. degree. But, the changes were made under the pressure of events, and, except for residency training, the trends in the lengthening and the shortening of the curriculum were not directly related to the educational needs of the different career objectives of the medical student. It is time that they were.

In the proposed plan, the total duration of each pathway through college, medical school, and hospital will no longer be arbitrarily fixed but will depend upon the curriculum content needed to qualify the student for his chosen career. As a result, the medical educational pathways will be of varying duration. Some will be longer than others. The student will know that the time required for his medical education was not arbitrarily fixed but was determined directly by his educational needs. Moreover, the feckless and endless discussion on the number of years required for a medical education will be ended once and for all. Finally, physicians will be graduated and will enter practice without any waste of time just as soon as they meet the formally established educational requirements.

G. **Qualifications for Admission to Medical Education**

Three points deserve special emphasis in regard to admission of students to be educated for the medicine of the future. One is the need for congruence between the requirements for admission and the content of each of the proposed curricular pathways of medical education. The second is to make sure that disadvantaged students may and do compete on equal terms for admission to medical education. Finally, large numbers of students in the general physician channel will have to be educated without compromising the basic and applied research programs and the other educational responsibilities of the medical school.

Assuming a set of uninterrupted curricular pathways from college matriculation until the end of hospital training, a provisional decision for acceptance of the student for medical education will have to be made at the time of college admission. Moreover, the student with clear-cut career objectives will have the advantage of matriculation at an early age in a curricular pathway specially designed for his needs. Since it is obvious that the kind of student aspiring to a career in molecular medical biology is different from one hoping to be a surgical specialist or a general physician, admission requirements will have to be tailored to each of the curricular pathways. It would be silly to select students for many widely different careers on the basis of a single set of qualifications. Admission requirements must, therefore, be established for each specific pathway. Students without defined career objectives at time of college admission would be accepted on the basis of the criteria for admission to the neutral channel. Most important, this proposed plan assures that students who have made an early career decision will be given the opportunity to pursue their special goals, while the undecided are given an opportunity to explore.

There remains the difficult task for the faculty to set up admission criteria for relatively young students for each of the medical care pathways. Tentative admission criteria to each pathway will have to be established, carefully studied, and then modified and classified as experience is accumulated. Selection of medical students at a relatively early age will not be as difficult as would at first appear. Indeed, we have a precedent. It has been demonstrated in countries with excellent basic and clinical medical research and medical care, for example, the Scandinavian countries and the United Kingdom, that students can be selected in their late teens for a medical career.

Even though firm decisions on final acceptance for a medical education will often be hard to make at the time of college matriculation, the unusually competent or incompetent student will be identified very early in his college career. For the rest, it will be necessary to watch and compare the students carefully during the early years of college education. This should not be difficult because, except for the more esoteric curricular pathways such as molecular medical biology and bioengineering, which should attract the unusual student who can be evaluated on more objective criteria, the differences in curriculum in the beginning portions of the various pathways will be relatively minor. Evaluation will also be possible at the time when the students who have elected the neutral pathway decide to shift to a specific one. Student competence can also be judged when they choose to move from one specific pathway to another or, indeed, may be forced to change pathways because of their inability to compete with other students having the same career objective. Admission requirements could be fitted to curricular pathways and career objectives, and the validity of student selection for particular medical careers could be determined early in the curriculum.

It must be made possible for intrinsically competent disadvantaged students, to compete for medical school admission on equal terms with their more fortunate colleagues. But in so doing, high standards must be maintained and the disadvantaged student accepted for medical education must be able to keep up with his class. In the long run, the disadvantaged student will not be favored by the recent tendency to apply admission criteria unevenly, or to establish arbitrary quotas to favor the admission of one variety or another of disadvantaged applicant. That trend can lead only to the disgraceful situation where less competent students are admitted by discriminating against the more competent ones.

If one accepts the concept that the major social responsibility of the medical school is to educate the best doctors for research and practice so as to give the best possible medical care to everybody, there can be no compromise with excellence. In the past when excellence was compromised, all kinds of reasons were found to admit less competent students. One has only to examine the history of medical education in Nazi Germany, the preference in medical school admission given in Eastern European countries to children of workers or peasants and to young activist members of the Communist Party, the university program in the People's Republic of China immediately after the cultural revolution, the veterans' preference in the Civil Service appointment of health department physicians, and the political biases in choosing high governmental medical or public health officials, to recognize the bankruptcy of a policy that selects and educates on criteria other than scientific and professional excellence. These examples are not farfetched. The zealots who furthered those programs were as fully convinced of the righteousness of their cause as are those who, for "social reasons" now urge preferential admission to medical school of certain groups of students on criteria other than excellence. If improvement of medical care is to proceed at an optimal rate, we dare not stoop to such practices.

But our society does have a responsibility to provide assistance to members of disadvantaged groups so that they can compete fairly for medical school admission. A few such programs are already under way. For example, it is possible for competent disadvantaged students educated at relatively inadequate colleges to be admitted to the Harvard Careers Summer Program[5] and obtain additional premedical education at Harvard College to make up for the deficiencies in their educational experience so that they may be better qualified for admission to medical school and be able to keep pace with their future classmates. Such programs are a good beginning but need to be extended and expanded. They meet an immediate need but must be supplemented by programs to increase the proportion of disadvantaged students applying to medical school. An integral part of this program is the upgrading of elementary schools and high schools for disadvantaged students.

In order to create a more thoroughgoing program at

5. R. S. Blacklow, "A Cooperative Educational Effort," *Harvard Medical Alumni Bulletin* 47 (September-October 1972): pp. 24–28.

an earlier student age, a national medical scholarship competition open to all disadvantaged high school students aspiring to a medical career should be established. Such a program has been long recommended in parallel with the Westinghouse Science Talent Search. Those successful in the competition should be supported in accordance with need until they are ready to enter their medical careers, as long as defined qualifications and standards continue to be met. The American Foundation for Negro Affairs (AFNA) has recently developed a program in Philadelphia "to recruit, retrain and support black and other minority students through a corridor of educational and clinical science activities directly leading to the biomedical careers." [6] The proportion of disadvantaged students in the pool of medical school applicants would thereby be increased. Medical students would then be selected from this larger pool of applicants using excellence as the major criterion. Thus, in the proposed total program of aiding disadvantaged applicants and increasing the size of the total pool, both aims would be accomplished. There would be greater opportunities for the disadvantaged student to enter medical education while high standards of medical research, education, and care could be maintained and improved.

Finally, the decision by the medical faculty to educate enough general physicians to meet the needs of a national health program must be reflected in admission policy and practice. Every effort will have to be made to

6. M. A. Bartley, "The Developing AFNA Plan: New Access Routes to Medical Careers," *Journal of the National Medical Association* (May 1972): pp. 264–267.

attract students to this career. Moreover, additional financial resources will have to be earmarked for the new program. It will be essential to convince governmental and other sources of funds that the general physician program must be supported by new funds and not by a diversion of financial support from other essential functions of the university medical school. Above all, the new program must not interfere with the traditional responsibility for the conduct of basic and applied laboratory and clinical research to expand the fund of medical knowledge. Medical leaders must have the wisdom to recognize that the new program should not bog down in competition between proponents of these two essential functions. Indeed, the better the collaboration among all medical leaders representing the entire spectrum of different points of view, the more likely it will be that human health will be improved in the future.

H. **Awarding of Degrees**

The change from a single medical curriculum to a set of different educational experiences must eventually be reflected in the specific recognition of accomplishment implicit in the awarding of university degrees. Indeed, the medical degrees to be granted in the proposed program will have to be congruent with each curricular pathway. The recent blossoming of combined M.D.-Ph.D. programs for students seeking a career in medical research is indicative of this new trend and suggests a simple and a practical solution.

Assuming a single, uninterrupted curriculum in each educational channel, the bachelor's degree could be awarded to all students in all pathways at the end of an arbitrary time period as is now done at the end of four years in most integrated college-medical school programs. The degree of Doctor of Medicine or Doctor of Dental Medicine would be awarded to all students in all pathways at the end of the medical school stage of the medical curriculum since local licensure laws will probably require a medical degree prior to internship or residency in the teaching hospital. But clearcut university responsibility for the entire sweep of the medical curriculum at all levels would be affirmed by granting to each graduate on successful completion of requirements at the end of his period of formal hospital training a supplementary degree testifying to his mastery of his individual curricular pathway. Later, if universities would agree on a system of external examiners, these specific degrees could be made equivalent to specialists' qualifications. Finally, this new method of awarding medical degrees should do away with our irresponsible system of state medical licensure in which each holder of an M.D. degree, who passes the state examination or its equivalent, is legally qualified to practice any or all specialties of medicine regardless of his personal competence. It is to be hoped that this new special degree will become a requirement for specialty licensure in all states.

The Curriculum for the General Physician

The principles governing the details of the curriculum for the general physician were outlined in a previous publication.[7] Since they would be of relatively little interest to

7. D. D. Rutstein, "Physicians for Americans: Two Medical Curricula: A New Proposal," *Lancet* 1 (March 4, 1961): pp. 498–501.

the nonprofessional reader, they are omitted from this text. For those interested, an abstract of the relevant portions of the article is published in the appendix to this book.

The Quality of Medical Care

12

Since medical care is concerned with the prevention and treatment of disease, improvement in its quality should be reflected in better health of the population served. This statement is straightforward enough. But without either a definition or a method for its measurement, the word "quality" has little meaning. A major objective of this book is to demonstrate that the quality of medical care can be measured. It will also become evident that measurements of quality must become the reference point in medical care research and the guiding light in the design and operation of a national health program, the critical determining factor in decisions to inaugurate, expand, contract, or terminate specific services.

The quality of medical care must be carefully differentiated from the efficiency of medical care. Both are very important but they must not be confused. Quality is the output of the "medical care machine" in the form of better health, while efficiency has to do with how well the individual parts of the machine perform their functions and at what cost. To be sure, if efficiency is increased, the quality of care may often be improved. But since this is not necessarily the case, improvement in quality has to be verified by direct measurement.

The most practical measurement of quality can be estimated from indices of unnecessary disease, unnecessary disability, and unnecessary untimely death. These terms are to be defined, measured, and used in their broadest context. Disease includes physical, mental, and social malfunction. Disability extends from physical paralysis to the inability for health reasons to hold a job or stay out of jail. Death is untimely when it strikes anyone who is or has the potential to be individually or socially productive. The occurrence in a particular area or population of unnecessary disease, such as measles, or unnecessary disability, such as unusable joints from contracted muscles following an accident, or unnecessary untimely death, such as death during childhood from lead poisoning, would provide evidence that the quality of medical care is not up to standard. Although some will object that health is more than the absence of illness, there are no quantitative positive ways to measure it at the present time. It will be demonstrated that the negative indices of unnecessary disease, disability, and untimely death can be measured in the population as a whole, and that they can be used as practical indices of the quality of medical care and of the health of the population.

In contrast with quality, efficiency can be measured in terms of the medical care machine, or its subunits, including the reliability and rapidity of laboratory services, the time required for admission of a patient to the hospital, the qualifications of professional personnel, the relative cost-effectiveness of substituting a practical nurse for a registered nurse in taking and in recording the temperature, pulse, and respiration of a patient, and of substituting a physician's assistant to perform certain tasks that do not demand the competence of the physician. In a word, quality measures the objectives of medical care, while efficiency is concerned with evaluation of the routes by which those objectives are reached.

As background for a program of the measurement of the quality and the efficiency of medical care, let us examine existing medical personnel standards, current institutional efforts to improve care and to protect their patient population, and present general population indices of medical care and health.

Existing Standards, Procedures, and Indices of Health and Medical Care

Qualifications of Medical Personnel

Many standards and procedures have been introduced to maintain and upgrade the qualifications of medical and allied medical personnel and to eliminate quackery. Universities are authorized by their charters to establish requirements for the granting of medical degrees. Qualifications have been fixed for the certification of physician specialists. Physicians and members of most of the allied medical professions have to pass licensure examinations in order to be permitted to practice. Professional organizations such as the American College of Surgeons, the American College of Physicians, and the College of General Practitioners, and comparable groups of the individual allied medical professions have membership requirements, have set up postgraduate educational obligations, and have initiated studies to help practitioners maintain their competence and keep up-to-date on important developments in their own fields. Even if all of these personnel standards and procedures were unquestionably beneficial, they might increase efficiency, but they do not, in themselves, guarantee that medical care provided to the patient will be of high quality, nor do they assure that the health of the population served will automatically be improved.

More recently, peer review, that is, evaluation of the practice of an individual physician by a group of his colleagues, has been introduced to help him toe the mark of established medical practice. But peer review is almost always in response to a complaint by the patient or the government of overcharging, or documentation by a hospital committee of overutilization of hospital beds by a physician; and not because of the "poor quality of the medical care." Moreover, in the past, physicians, as is true for practically every group of human beings, have been almost totally unsuccessful in policing themselves. Every county medical society is charged with maintaining the highest professional, ethical, and moral standards of its members. But what have medical societies done about physicians caught in Medicaid scandals, or what have they done to develop programs to prevent recurrence of such scandals? The answer is, Very little. Peer review has recently evolved into "medical foundations" under the aegis of organized medicine and has led to the congressional legislation that created the Professional Standards Review Organization.[1] The kinds of data that they are proposing to collect may relate to the efficiency and the cost of medical care but will not provide direct information about its quality.

Institutional Medical Care

Many kinds of standards and methods of evaluation have been established to upgrade hospital services. The Commission on Hospital Accreditation does appraise such institutional attributes as the appropriateness of administrative policies, the qualifications of governing boards and management, the acceptance of professional responsibility by the medical staff, the safety of its environmental services including fire protection, the standards of the practice of pathology and pharmaceutics, the adequacy of the social services, and the completeness, appropriateness, and availability of the medical record. Unquestionably, the Commission has been successful in eliminating marginal and substandard institutions. Moreover, voluntary health agencies, such as the American Cancer Society and the American Heart Association, have published standards for specialty hospital clinics and have defined diagnostic criteria for such diseases as rheumatic fever and certain malignant tumors.

Most of these standards and regulations to upgrade the organizational structure and the physical plant of the hospital are really concerned with the efficiency of the

1. C. E. Welch, "Professional Standards Review Organization—Problems and Prospects," *New England Journal of Medicine* 289 (August 9, 1973): pp. 291–295.

methods of providing medical care. Most of them do not measure outcome in the form of better health of the treated population and are, therefore, not directly concerned with the quality of care received by the institutional population. This conclusion is not surprising, given the current but avoidable difficulty of defining hospital populations and the geographical areas from which they come, and of following hospital patients for long enough periods of time to tell what actually happens to them.

Nevertheless, there are some measurements that do examine the effect of institutional medical care on the health of the patient population. The best known of the practices designed to measure, protect, and improve the health of hospital patients are clinical research studies that make direct measurements of outcome. For example, control studies of such specific therapies as highly specialized surgical procedures or new drugs do make a precise estimate of their effects on the health of the treated patients. The results of such studies, when successful, influence the practice of other physicians within the research hospital and in other institutions, and improve the outcome of their patients. Another example is the routine examination in most hospitals of all tissues removed at operation to determine whether the surgery was justified. In some hospitals this routine practice has been expanded to the monitoring of deaths and recovery rates subsequent to specific surgical procedures, and the results and side effects of drug therapy. Finally, and most important, in some hospitals the records of all patients who die are currently reviewed by the chief of staff with the visiting and resident physicians and the interns responsible for their care, to identify the preventable deaths in order to guide future hospital practice and to avoid the recurrence of the same kind of mistakes. Unfortunately, in most hospitals this valuable procedure is either neglected or is conducted in a perfunctory manner.

We still have a long way to go in evaluating the quality of institutional care. We cannot yet assess the effect of a hospital's care on the outcome of all of its patients. We must devise methods of estimating the quality of hospital care, not only in fatal cases, but also in serious nonfatal, disabling, recurrent, and even in run-of-the-mill diseases. The establishment of a national health program will simplify this task. In the Scandinavian countries and the United Kingdom and in the Kaiser-Permanente Program in the United States, a necessary ingredient of the fiscal operation of a health service is a computerized, itemized record of the costs of each procedure conducted on every person insured in the program. Thus the essential facts necessary for the monitoring of the patient's health and for assuring continuity of care, if already built into the accounting record, make it possible to ascertain, for example, the results of specific therapies and the outcome of specific illnesses in defined populations. This is in contrast with our lack of system where patient follow-up in most hospitals for most diseases is extremely awkward and where the effect of specific therapy on the eventual outcome may be almost impossible to ascertain. The development of specially designed and uniform records with due regard to preserving confidentiality for the patient and to protecting the physician against lawsuits would increase acceptance of a quality-control program by the medical profession and could do much to simplify the extremely difficult problem of determining whether patients had received optimal care in a hospital.

It must now be clear that procedures that evaluate and improve the efficiency of the individual components of a system of institutional care, including its administration, personnel, resources, and services, are different from those that measure outcome as an index of the quality of care provided to the patients. This is not to say that measures of efficiency of medical care are unimportant. Nursing time must not be wasted. Laboratory services must be rapid, precise, and provided at minimal cost. Patient and physician waiting time must be kept to a minimum. Professional competence must be high. Duplication in superspecialist facilities, such as open heart surgical services, radiation tratment centers, and coronary and intensive care units must be eliminated. Hospital beds must be saved for those patients who really need them. There must be a close, personal physician-patient relationship to further acceptance of recommended medical procedures and to encourage and reassure the patient. This is particularly important in the myriad of minor illnesses that, although not life-threatening, may seriously incapacitate the patient. Constant surveillance and special studies at national and regional levels, using well-established methods, are necessary to assure that all parts of the medical care machine operate at top efficiency and at minimal cost in money and personnel. An administrative mechanism must be developed and be in operation in every hospital to maintain efficiency at the highest possible level.

Let us now concentrate on the more difficult problem of evaluation of the quality of medical care within an institution. The quality of institutional care may not be improved, even if all efficiency measures have been built into the system, since they do not necessarily guarantee better health to anyone served by the program. Moreover, the best quality of medical care keeps some people out of hospital beds. Therefore, statistics derived only from institutionalized patients are not by themselves adequate measures of quality. All measurements of institutional efficiency and productivity and their implementation must be supplemented by direct measures of the quality of medical care, that is, the output of the medical care machine, as reflected in the level of unnecessary disease, disability, and untimely death in the total population served. Such measurements are essential if we are to establish a priority listing of individual health procedures and programs, both within the hospital and outside its walls, as reflected by the level of health in the community. This recommended procedure, although revolutionary for the total gamut of therapeutic medicine, is not new. It has long been followed in preventive programs as, for example, when a vaccine is introduced to eliminate a communicable disease such as poliomyelitis or diphtheria. After immunization programs are instituted, the population is monitored for the occurrence of cases of the preventable disease.

Indices of Health in the General Population

Let us examine the validity of the two most commonly used indices of health of the general population: life expectancy and infant mortality.[2] Life expectancy at birth is a theoretical estimate in a particular year of the average length of life of a newborn baby.[3] It takes into account the potential burden of all fatal illnesses throughout an entire lifetime. Life expectancy is a useful comparative measuring stick of the impact of mortality on a total population. It provides leads to studies and to treatments that could decrease the burden of fatal illness on a population. A study of a population with a shortened life expectancy should reveal an excess of those illnesses in which mortality can be prevented, such as tuberculosis, malaria, and the diarrheal diseases of early childhood.

Life expectancy does have its limitations as an index of health. It is concerned with life and death but does not reflect the occurrence of illness or disability in the living population. Moreover, it does not evaluate the productivity of those who are alive in that a person actively working, for example, is counted as the same as a senile patient of the same age in a nursing home. In a word, the life expectancy index does not reflect the quality of life. Nevertheless, the index does have value if carefully used, but it has to be supplemented by other more specific indices of health.

The second index, the infant mortality rate, is the number of infants who die in their first year of life out of every thousand who are born alive. Infant mortality is a

2. D. D. Rutstein, *The Coming Revolution in Medicine* (Cambridge, Massachusetts: MIT Press, 1967): pp. 11–28.

3. Life expectancy of a newborn baby in a particular year is calculated on the assumption that he would be exposed throughout his lifetime to the age-specific mortality rates for that year.

sensitive indicator of the effectiveness of medicine in the social structure and of the guidance offered to the public by the medical profession. The infant mortality rate can be decreased by improved living and sanitation standards, by better maternal and obstetrical care, by adequate nutrition, and by more careful pediatric supervision and medical care during the first year of life. In a sense, this index is an expression of what a society, under the guidance of its physicians, will do for its mothers and babies. Living conditions and nutrition must be improved wherever possible. But the effect of these factors on the infant mortality rate does not support the inference that many babies' lives cannot be saved by better medical care. Indeed, a study in 1970 of the Massachusetts Medical Society[4] demonstrated that 35 percent of a random sample of infant deaths within that state were preventable by medical means.

But infant mortality, like life expectancy, is only a measure of death. It is not an index of infant growth and development, does not identify the incidence or prevalence of nonfatal disease, and is not a measure of disability in childhood. Nevertheless, major differences in infant mortality in nations, states, and local regions, and in racial, economic, and other population groups have pointed up remediable deficiencies in medical care. Changing time trends in this index have also called attention to specific triumphs and failures in the improvement of human health.

4. D. M. Muirhead, "Report on Perinatal and Infant Mortality in Massachusetts, 1967 and 1968," Committee on Perinatal Welfare of the Massachusetts Medical Society (December 1971).

Although life expectancy and infant mortality are crude and incomplete indices of the health of the population, they are infinitely better than the undocumented statements of medical pundits testifying periodically to the excellence of the health of the population of the United States. But we do need to take better aim with more specific and sensitive indices of the nation's health. We must create new indices that will focus specifically on our preventable and remediable health problems. A beginning has been made by the Center for Disease Control in the creation of such health indices as prematurity statistics, the percentage of a given age group with anemia, measles attack rates, and the percentage of entering school children who have positive tuberculin tests. Indices such as these promise to provide guidance to health programs in the future.

Whatever the system of measuring the output of the medical care system in the form of better health, we must begin by counting those health events that can be identified, quantified, and classified. At first, we will be limited to the identification of undesirable health events, that is, the frequency of unnecessary disease, disability, and untimely death as negative indices of the quality of care provided to the population served. The proposed quality control system will be criticized because it cannot in the beginning quantify the positive and some of the more subtle and personal aspects of health. Moreover, it will be difficult at first to correlate social, environmental, and economic causes directly with specific types of unnecessary disease, disability, and untimely death. But just as the investigation of an airplane accident goes beyond the immediate reasons for the crash to the implications of the design, method of manufacture, maintenance, and operation of the plane, so will the study of undesirable, unnecessary health events yield crucial information on those scientific, medical, social, and personal factors that could lead to better health. Eventually, we will define positive factors that can be measured directly. Moreover, the evidence collected will not be limited to those factors that yield only to medical measures of control. If there is clear-cut evidence that identifiable social, environmental, economic, or genetic factors are responsible for special varieties of disease, disability, or untimely death, these will be pinpointed and eliminated whenever possible. Above all, we must stop guessing and go to work. We must start *immediately* to measure and eradicate those unnecessary undesirable events that significantly impair the health of our country. To accomplish this, let us now turn to the development and implementation of a feasible quality control system.

Quality Control Systems 13

Two different kinds of control systems will be needed to collect, analyze, and feed back those data on the quality of care that are essential to the administration of an effective national health program, designed to bring all potential health benefits to all of our people: a *guidance system* to measure, follow, and interpret accomplishments and failures, and to lay out a course for future programs; and an *early warning system* to identify sudden outcroppings of undesirable health events that may demand immediate action. Both systems will be focused on the occurrence of unnecessary disease, disability, and untimely death as negative indices of the quality of care. The *guidance system* will determine and compare their statistical distribution throughout the country and in each medical care region, while the *early warning system* will signal and evaluate the epidemiological occurrence of individual sentinel health events.

The Guidance System

The guidance system will serve as a mechanism for the immediate and continuous evaluation of national and regional health. The data collected on unnecessary disease, disability, and untimely death should aid in the planning of health programs, should identify specific successes and failures, should pinpoint remedial action for the improvement of health and for the better treatment of patients and should be channeled into a feedback loop of information to guide those responsible for the direction of the program.

The immediate and continuous evaluation of national and regional health to supply a constant stream of relevant and reliable information to guide the program will require that:

• Data collection in the guidance system must begin at the earliest moment in order to establish a base line for national and regional health prior to the inauguration of a national health program. Moreover, the earlier the data are collected, the more useful they will be in the actual planning for a national health program. These objectives will be all the more easily accomplished if the guidance system can make use of existing data-collection agencies and research programs.

• The measurements made must be representative of the population to be served by the program. The sample of individuals studied must be representative for all factors that are known to have a significant effect on health, including age, sex, race, geography, and such social influences as economics and environment. In a word, the data collected on disease, disability, and untimely death

must fairly represent the actual health status of the population served.
• Assuming a regional system of medical care in any carefully designed national health program, it will be essential that comparable data be collected on an adequate and representative sample of the whole country and of each medical care region in order to identify the unusual accomplishments and the preventable failures in the nation and in each region. With such information, it becomes possible to introduce modifications that would have an immediate and direct effect on the health of individuals within the region.
• Measurements must be reproducible and comparable over time in order to discern and evaluate trends in national and regional health for continuous guidance of the program.
• A high priority must be placed on the collection of those specific items of data yielded by interview questions, examination procedures, and laboratory tests that are most relevant and sensitive to the identification of preventable and remediable health conditions and that can be used as indices of health. Initially, a thorough medical evaluation of human illnesses will establish a tentative list of unnecessary diseases and disabilities, and causes of untimely deaths. Eventually, continuous re-examination of the usefulness of the data collected on those diseases that are preventable or are better treated early than late, on the disabilities that can be forestalled, and on the untimely deaths that ought not to have occurred should result in the collection of the kinds of data and the creation of the specific health indices that

are most relevant to the maintenance of the health of a maximum number of individuals in the population.

There are many ways in which the guidance system could be related to the care of the individual. For example, the guidance system could be of great assistance in the design and implementation of screening programs for the detection, as early as possible, of previously unrecognized cases of diseases that are better treated early than late. As an example, let us examine the factors affecting the occurrence of cancer of the uterine cervix to guide the design of a screening program to identify early cases and to prevent deaths from this disease. Recent epidemiologic and laboratory evidence suggests that cancer of the cervix results from viral infection (Herpes II Virus) transmitted during sexual intercourse. The disease is very common in prostitutes and rare in nuns, and is more frequent in women with a history of early intercourse, early marriage, and exposure to multiple sexual partners. The occurrence of the illness may often be heralded by bleeding between periods but it can be suspected, before symptoms and before invasion of adjacent tissue, by a Papanicolaou screening test. Treatment at that stage of this disease is curative. Ideally, screening programs should begin after first intercourse. Practically, the program should be inaugurated as a part of the premarital examination and be repeated at each pregnancy and after each delivery, and be performed at least once a year. Such a program should cut the death rate from cancer of the cervix to very low levels.

The yields of screening programs for most such diseases in the general population are usually so small as to be wasteful of medical manpower and money. Given the diseases that justify screening, the guidance system would reveal and identify high-risk populations where the yield should justify the effort. Tuberculosis is a classic example. The current national incidence and prevalence of this disappearing disease does not justify general population screening with tuberculin tests or by x-ray. But tuberculosis does have a relatively high incidence in special population groups such as family contacts of known cases and reported deaths, and in low income groups such as agricultural workers, and recently urbanized populations, for example, Puerto Ricans. The guidance system could pinpoint the specific groups where the highest yield might be expected. Furthermore, there must be close liaison between the guidance system and those responsible for screening programs so that the former would know which diseases to look for and the latter could conduct their screening on populations of highest risk. Finally, there must be continuous feedback from the screening program to the medical care program so that on discovery of a case, the patient would be treated immediately.

The guidance system must have a research component to improve its day-to-day operation and to identify leads that deserve intensive research. The data collection system must constantly take advantage of all medical discoveries anywhere in the world that identify new categories of unnecessary disease, disability, and untimely death. Thus, for example, if a new and highly effective therapy of cancer of the breast were discovered, survey questions and examination procedures would have to be modified to pinpoint the unnecessary cases and deaths from this disease so that it could serve as another indicator of the quality of care.

The analysis of the collected data in the guidance system must be designed to identify significant leads that deserve intensive research. It is unlikely that the National Center for Health Statistics, which would be responsible for operation of the guidance system, will have the scientific resources to study in depth the research leads emerging from its wide-ranging statistical surveys. There must be a mechanism to relate the extensive statistical research of the guidance system to the intensive basic laboratory and clinical research activities in our medical schools and in their teaching hospitals, that is, the central hospitals of the proposed regional system. The Medical Research Council of Great Britain, which has been very successful in relating the extensive national vital statistics to intensive research programs in universities in the United Kingdom, can be used as a model. In the United States, the Center for Disease Control through its laboratories, its epidemiologic surveillance resources, and its network of sentinel hospitals could play the same role as the Medical Research Council does in Great Britain. In the quality control system, the Center for Disease Control could also make on-the-spot investigations of any outcroppings of unnecessary disease, disability, or untimely death revealed by the surveys of the National Center for Health Statistics. The National Center for Health Statistics and the Center for Disease Control in the Department of Health, Education, and Welfare are already conducting programs that with minor modifications to focus on preventable and remediable health conditions could perform all of the functions for which they would be responsible as outlined in the quality control system in this blueprint.

Let us examine the many ways in which interrelated research could add significantly to the knowledge now yielded by independent extensive and intensive research units. A productive lead could emerge from either kind of research. Let us demonstrate by examples from the Medical Research Council how investigative leads that emerge from analysis of *extensive* population data yield important health information when subjected to *intensive* controlled research. It was discovered in a Medical Research Council study, that the sudden increase in mortality among young asthmatic patients revealed by death certificate analysis correlated with the uncontrolled overuse of new powerful inhalation drugs that dilate the bronchial tubes and relieve asthmatic attacks. Unfortunately, when large doses are inhaled, the lungs become nonreactive and the patient may die. As a result of this discovery, control of inhalation therapy prevented unnecessary untimely deaths. Another study by the Medical Research Council documented the suspicion aroused by the large number of cases reported to the Committee on Safety of Drugs that women taking oral contraceptives were subject to an excess risk of blood-clotting complications. Indeed, this conclusion was found subsequently to be compatible with the increase of deaths from this cause.

Conversely, a lead may be revealed by *intensive* research that will require an *extensive* research study for its validation. The development of poliomyelitis vaccine followed this route. The laboratory discovery that polio virus could be so changed that upon injection it would immunize the individual without making him sick with the disease required the extensive Francis and other field trials for both Salk and Sabin vaccine in order to justify their efficacy and safety in the population at large.

Integration of intensive and extensive research is now so well accepted as to be almost routine in the prevention of obviously epidemic illnesses such as the acute infectious diseases. This combined approach is beginning to be generally introduced in research in such chronic diseases as cancer, heart disease, or mental illness where the epidemiologic implications are more subtle. It must, however, be clear that large scale epidemiologic surveys or clinical trials will require specially organized research units, either as supplements to the guidance system or on an ad hoc basis as in the Francis field trial, and will be greatly facilitated by the proposed system of individual complete medical records.

An integrated extensive-intensive research program could also be applied to noninfectious diseases. There is, for example, a strong belief that the apparently increased occurrence of disseminated lupus, a serious illness, has resulted from the rapidly expanding use of some of the recently discovered chemotherapeutic or antibiotic drugs such as sulfadiazine. This suspicion cannot be effectively explored separately either by an extensive statistical epidemiological research unit or by an intensive laboratory or clinical research team. The extensive population study unit could obtain crude survey data on the distribution of cases and deaths from the disease, and on the distribution of suspected drugs in the population at large from the pattern of prescription sales. The clinical and laboratory investigators could by direct testing determine which drug would precipitate an exacerbation of the disease in individual patients or would initiate or augment the derangements of immunity that characterize this illness. But such experiments on human patients are unethical.

A joint effort by both groups would probably yield a definitive answer to this crucial question. The clinical and laboratory investigators could assist the statisticians and epidemiologists in precise case finding and in the identification and evaluation of the effects of the suspected chemotherapeutic agents or antibiotics in patients who have been treated with them for other reasons. In turn, statistical and epidemiological surveys and case-finding programs could guide the clinical and laboratory investigators to those individuals who deserve intensive study where the drugs in question have been repeatedly used, for example, sulfa drugs in those who have had urinary infection. The two kinds of investigators, working together, could devise and conduct a well-controlled experiment so that the clinical impression of a drug-disease relationship could be affirmed or denied in a long-range population study in a sample large enough to yield significant results.

In practical terms, the implementation of the proposed joint research effort will depend upon the creation of a population laboratory affiliated with the central teaching hospital of each medical care region. At present, our haphazard medical care makes it most difficult to define the population served by the average large teaching hospital. But a great advantage of the proposed national health program is that the total population of the region would become, by definition, the total population served by the central hospital affiliated with a medical school. The study population in the region could be selected by the National Center for Health Statistics and could be a part of one of its probability survey populations. As a result, national and regional data would be comparable.

This national-regional compatible data collection system could have a major impact on health. It would become possible to compare the health status of the regions with one another and with the level of national health. Such objective comparison would become a major basis for affirmative decisions for repairing the gaps in services and improving the medical care of the population in a particular region or in the nation as a whole. The same data collection system could identify unnecessary undesirable health events produced by environmental factors such as malnutrition, occupational hazards, and poor housing.

The national-regional system would have another beneficial effect. Theoretically, human biological studies should have general application to entire populations of sick patients. But only too often, the patients studied, because of the way they are selected—patients admitted to a hospital or fatal cases on which an autopsy has been performed, for example—usually represent only the more severely ill patients in a subgroup of the disease. The classic example is hypertension, where the observations on very sick patients in a hospital may or may not be applicable to the large number of individuals in the general population suffering from high blood pressure of all degrees of severity. In the proposed population laboratory, appropriate samples of patients who have a particular illness could be selected for specific biological studies, the results of which could be clearly applicable and helpful both to the subjects and to the patients in the defined segment of the total illness.

All in all, the contributions of an integrated extensive-intensive research program could be electrifying. Research discoveries in the study sample population of the hospital in each region could have immediate significance for regional and for national health. In turn, the research findings in national epidemiological surveys could accelerate and support intensive research in the local study population and be immediately applicable for the medical care of the total population of the region.

Thus, it is time for the meticulous microscopic view of the basic laboratory and clinical investigator to be brought into focus with the less detailed but more comprehensive telescopic field of vision of the epidemiologist. Each will obtain a new insight into his problems when they are viewed in the perspective of the other kind of investigator. The laboratory and clinical investigator probing his problem in depth would obtain a window to the world as he sees how his discoveries relate to the total constellation of illness and to the population at large. In turn, the epidemiologist will make his observations in sharper resolution if his findings are subject to meticulous controlled investigation in the laboratory and in the clinic. Some problems are solved by studying the energy emitted by a star. Others are clarified by the definition of the structure and movement of entire galaxies. But for a fuller understanding of the universe of health and disease, the knowledge yielded by both kinds of scientific endeavor must be closely interrelated so that they can be brought together into the same focus.

Implementation of the Guidance System
Let us examine and analyze our existing medical data collection resources and then indicate how they could be modified and supplemented in order to become an effective guidance system for a national program. It is, indeed, fortunate that the collection of extensive, precise, and reproducible data already under way in the National Center for Health Statistics of the United States Department of Health, Education, and Welfare provides an excellent base for the development of a guidance system for a national health program. During the past fifteen years, an extensive national system of collection and analysis of data concerning disease, disability, and death has been developed. With minor modifications in program the Center could change its focus and concentrate on *unnecessary* disease, disability, and untimely death. Let us examine the potential contribution of the Center for each of these parameters separately, identify other data collection resources, and specify how their data could be integrated into a guidance system.

Unnecessary Disease
The National Center for Health Statistics obtains continuous information on the current distribution of disease

throughout the country by two methods: the collection of household health data by direct interview, and the medical examination of individuals to obtain data on specifically defined diseases and conditions of ill health. Interviews are conducted weekly with representatives of a national probability sample of 800 U.S. households to obtain information on the occurrence of perceived illnesses and complaints. A different random sample of 800 households is interviewed each week so that every year such information is collected on more than 40,000 different households. In the second study, the Health and Nutrition Examination Survey, a medical examination is performed approximately every three years on every one of the more than 27,000 members of another random sample of the population of the United States. The more detailed data collected in the examination survey are, of course, not as current as those of the interview survey, but their greater precision provides a more complete view of the current health status of the population of the country. It will be necessary to change or modify questions on the interview forms and the procedures of the physical examination to focus more clearly on the occurrence of unnecessary disease and to meet special needs of a guidance system for a national health program. But it is clear that with minor modifications the machinery already exists for the collection of representative current information on the incidence and prevalence of unnecessary disease in the population of the United States.

In its turn, the Center for Disease Control in Atlanta, Georgia, collects from the fifty states, weekly reports of cases of most of the communicable diseases that occur in our country. Moreover, the Epidemic Intelligence Service of the Center, upon invitation from the states, makes intensive investigations of practically all of the important epidemics of communicable disease in the United States. These data on communicable diseases appropriately interrelated with the survey information could become an essential element in medical care guidance. Indeed, the pooling and integration of properly selected individual items of data collected by these two agencies could establish the status of and follow trends in frequencies of individual unnecessary diseases for the purposes of a guidance system of a national health program.

Unnecessary Disability

The National Center for Health Statistics in both the interview and the examination probability surveys elicits quantitative information on the kinds of partial and total physical disability—for example, chronic arthritis or chronic neurological or chronic heart disease—that limit the activities of individuals in our country. For the purposes of a national health program, it would become necessary to expand the surveys to include mental disability and to search for the underlying causes of disability in every case. When needed, such survey information could be supplemented by the data collected by the Social Security Administration on the number and kinds of diseases which cause the cases of total and permanent disability that qualify for financial support.

Unnecessary Untimely Death

The National Center for Health Statistics currently receives copies of all death certificates collected by all of the state health departments in the United States. To be sure, there is a wide variability in the quality of death certificate data. But, death certificates do contain the information on age and cause of death that is essential to preliminary estimates of untimely death in specified populations. If collaborative studies were conducted jointly by biostatisticians of the National Center for Health Statistics, the epidemiologists in the Center for Disease Control, and the intensive research workers in our medical school teaching hospitals, the scientific and medical reasons for many of the unnecessary untimely deaths revealed by death certificate analysis could be effectively determined. With such knowledge, it would become feasible to design and implement specific national and regional health programs for the saving of useful lives that are now being wasted. The classic successful example is the collaborative extensive and intensive maternal mortality studies of the New York Academy of Medicine that were followed by a sharp decrease in the maternal death rate in New York City in the 1930s.[1]

The National Center for Health Statistics also receives, on a current basis, copies of all birth certificates and fetal death certificates (beginning in the twentieth week of pregnancy) from all of the fifty states. Combined analysis of birth and death certificates provides the precise estimates of mortality in late pregnancy, at time of delivery, and in the first year of life—that is, fetal, neonatal, and infant death rates—needed to save the

1. New York Academy of Medicine, Committee on Public Health Relations, *Maternal Mortality in New York City. A Study of All Puerperal Deaths 1930–1932* (New York: The Commonwealth Fund, 1933).

lives of babies whose deaths are preventable. Once again, leads revealed by these statistical analyses could be explored with the Center for Disease Control and with research workers at the regional medical school.

Medical Resources and Flow Patterns of Disease, Disability, and Death

The National Center for Health Statistics has been conducting studies of the occurrence of disease, disability, and death at various stages of medical care and on the use of specified health facilities and resources. Thus, information is being collected on the distribution of disease and death in a representative sample of patients discharged from short-stay hospitals throughout the country. More recently, to help in resolving problems of care for chronically ill patients, a similar study was instituted on a random sample of nursing home populations. Now that the utter chaos of ambulatory care has created our greatest immediate medical care problem, the Center is initiating a study of disease, diagnosis, and treatment in a representative sample of ambulatory patients. These sets of data on the use of the different kinds of health resources combined with data on the distribution of unnecessary disease, disability, and untimely death should provide the basic information necessary for initial and continuing estimates of institutional, personnel, and economic needs of the national and of the regional health programs.

Feasibility of a Guidance System

It should be clear that with relatively minor modifications of existing research facilities it is feasible to develop

a reliable guidance system for a national health program. Indeed, the basic structure, flexibility of program, and accomplishments of the National Center for Health Statistics make it very likely that it could bring together and analyze the kinds of extensive data needed to measure the quality of medical care for the guidance of a national health program. But the precise collection and the effective use of the data in a guidance system will depend upon prior completion of the following prerequisites:
1. a clear statement of the objectives of a national health program;
2. precise operating definitions of the terms unnecessary disease, disability, and untimely death;
3. division of the country into medical care regions;
4. a recasting of the data collection system to evaluate health in each region and in the country as a whole;
5. continuous evaluation of each item of data for its relevance to national and regional health;
6. the creation of new more sensitive health indices of preventable and treatable conditions;
7. closer collaboration among the National Center for Health Statistics, the Center for Disease Control, and other statistical and epidemiological units, and the intensive, in-depth research programs of medical school teaching hospitals; and
8. a channel for the feedback of critical health information to those responsible for the guidance of the medical care program.

If the above conditions are satisfied, a guidance system to

control and improve the quality of health could be highly effective in an efficient national health program.

The Early Warning System

To supplement the *guidance system* in maintaining the quality of medical care, there is a need for an *early warning system* to identify sudden unwarranted episodes of ill health that demand immediate action for their control. At the present state of medical science, knowledge, and resources, there are dramatic, immediately recognizable sentinel cases or groups of cases of disease, disability, and untimely death that simply should not take place or should occur only at or below a predetermined level. When they do take place, in order to prevent similar events in the future, we must search for the underlying reasons just as we do after airplane crashes.

There are many examples of such sentinel health events. In a country that is said to have "adequate medical care" there should theoretically not be a single case of diphtheria, tetanus, measles, typohoid fever, or lead poisoning. The disability rate from paralytic poliomyelitis, bone rickets, or from occupational diseases such as silicosis should be zero. Ideally, there should not be a single death from unnecessary surgery, from tuberculosis, cancer of the uterine cervix, tumors resulting from asbestos inhalation, or from leukemia induced by exposure to ionizing radiation. There should be very few cases of German measles in early pregnancy and practically no disability from eye, brain, or heart defects, or from deafness in the offspring. Most patients with disabling rheumatoid arthritis need not become bedridden and permanent disability from fracture due to an accident should be rare. Death from Rh incompatibility in the newborn, from the diarrheal diseases of infancy, or from acute blood loss at any time of life should be uncommon. The death rate from Hodgkin's Disease, cancer of the lung, and cancer of the large bowel should remain below specified limits.

All these examples of sentinel health events could be recognized by an early warning system. The optimal asymptotes could almost be reached if everyone performed perfectly and everything went well. To be sure, in this imperfect world under the best of circumstances there will always be cases of preventable or curable disease, and disability, and some untimely deaths. But whenever such sentinel health events are identified by the guidance system, a practicing physician, or another member of the health care team, a newspaper reporter or any reliable source, they should be investigated and, if confirmed, the underlying causes must be ascertained and eliminated if recurrences of unnecessary disease, disability, or untimely death are to be prevented.

The early warning system would be implemented by the Center for Disease Control using the same surveillance system now used for the control of communicable diseases. A report of an outcropping of an unnecessary undesirable health event in the reports from the National Center for Health Statistics, a state health department, the Federal Health Board (chapter 14), a regional health board, or from any other reliable source would be subject

to epidemiological investigation to verify the report of the event, identify the mechanism responsible for its occurrence, control the outbreak, and prevent recurrences in the same geographic area and throughout the country. Fortunately, the Center for Disease Control is already undertaking such a program in a limited way in the surveillance of:
1. legal abortions for factors affecting morbidity and mortality;
2. cases of septicemia from contaminated commercially prepared intravenous fluids;
3. drug reactions, including the recently identified hepatitis associated with isoniazide treatment in tuberculous patients;
4. iron deficiency anemia in children in poverty areas; and
5. sentinel hospitals in early warning systems to identify such events as pathogenic bacteria resistant to antibiotics, and the inadequacy of commercial reagents used in bacteriological and other laboratory tests.

Thus, the Center for Disease Control is already organized to conduct and has trained personnel to implement an early warning system.

For the purposes of an early warning system, the Center for Disease Control would compile and maintain an up-to-date complete list of all of the kinds of reportable sentinel diseases, sentinel disabilities, and sentinel causes of untimely death for the use of all those members of national and regional health systems, including doctors, allied health personnel, statisticians, epidemiologists, and others whose work makes it possible for them to identify and to signal the occurrence of sentinel health events.

An operating branch of the early warning system would be established in each medical care region. A report of a sentinel health event would alert the regional health board to the possibility of a remediable defect in the local medical care system. The regional board would then be responsible for initiating steps to identify and repair the defect so as to ward off additional unnecessary cases of the disease or the disability, or needless untimely deaths.

It should be clear that the sole objective of an early warning system is to prevent the repeated recurrence of the same kinds of unnecessary disease, disability, and untimely death. The system would not be concerned with identifying incompetent physicians, fixing guilt, assessing criminal penalties, or instituting malpractice proceedings. These are the responsibilities of legally authorized administrative officials or the courts acting within the framework of the criminal law and of the malpractice acts, and not of the early warning system of a national medical care program. To be certain that the early warning system could not deviate from its sole objective but would maintain the reporting of sentinel events at a high level, it is essential that a confidential record system be established that will handle cases by number and assure anonymous reports.

Since the objective of the early warning system is to prevent the recurrence of each kind of sentinel health event, it is necessary to understand that the chain of responsibility for sentinel health events may be long and complex. Thus, the unnecessary case of diphtheria, measles, or poliomyelitis may be the responsibility of the physician who failed to immunize his patient, the medical society that opposed community clinics, the health officer who did not implement the program, the politician who failed to appropriate the needed funds, the religious views of the family, or the mother who didn't bother to bring her baby for immunization. The untimely death from typhoid fever, ionizing radiation, preventable poisoning, or occupational disease may result from legislative inaction, the lack of effective control of sanitary or environmental health hazards, or poor medical care by an uninformed, careless, or casual physician. Death from cancer of the lung may be due to the patient's unwillingness or inability to give up cigarette smoking, the reassuring statements put out by the advertiser or manufacturer of cigarettes or by the senator or congressman from a tobacco state, the absence of an effective health information program in the public schools and in the community, or more rarely from an error in diagnosis or from poor surgical care. Permanent crippling from chronic disabling diseases such as rheumatoid arthritis can be the result of inadequate medical management of the underlying disease, insufficient instruction and demonstration to the patient of an exercise regimen, lack of facilities for physiotherapy, or the unwillingness of the patient to cooperate in the never-ending struggle against frozen joints and contracted muscles. The reader may develop further examples for himself.

When, after careful study, the responsibility for a

particular sentinel health event is finally assigned on the basis of the particular errors of omission or commission that led to its occurrence, a recurrence of the same kind of event may or may not be preventable in the future. For example, it is likely that poor surgical care which may be responsible for a very tiny proportion of deaths from lung cancer could be improved. But the smoker who is "hooked" on cigarettes will, in all probability, be unable to break the habit that is responsible for the overwhelming majority of deaths from lung cancer. Thus, it is clear that the physician cannot be solely responsible for many of the errors of omission and commission that result in a sentinel health event.

Nevertheless, in every kind of unnecessary disease, disability, and untimely death, the physician himself has the initial and also some continuing responsibility. He is the only individual competent to provide the leadership and the professional guidance to the politician, the administrator, and the patient, to industry, and to the public. They may, of course, not take the physician's advice but that does not relieve him of the responsibility for the input of the scientific facts and the professional knowledge that are directly relevant to the improvement of human health and to the prevention of community decisions that may result in unnecessary disease, disability, and untimely death.

Let us examine the quality of medical care in the state of Texas in 1970, when much unnecessary tragedy could have been prevented if an early warning system had been in operation. In 1970—the same year when the miracles of heart transplantation in Houston were being advertised to the world—the largest diphtheria epidemic in several decades in the United States (201 cases and three deaths) was raging in San Antonio. Moreover, of the total of 34 cases of paralytic poliomyelitis in the United States in 1970, more than half—actually 24 cases—took place in the state of Texas. In that same year there was also a statewide epidemic of thousands of cases of measles—another completely preventable disease.

The potential impact of an early warning system is demonstrated dramatically by the measles outbreak in Texarkana, a city of 50,000 divided by the Texas-Arkansas boundary line and located in Miller County, Arkansas, and Bowie County, Texas.[2] The 633 reported cases of measles in that epidemic had a very curious distribution; 606 (95.7 percent) occurred in the 11,185 children age one to nine in Texas, while only 27 cases occurred in the 6,016 children in the same age group in the Arkansas part of town. As demonstrated in studies conducted by the Center for Disease Control, only 57 percent of the Texas children had immunity against measles in comparison with more than 95 percent of the Arkansas children. The underlying reason was obvious. Extensive measles immunization programs had been conducted in Arkansas, but consistent with long-standing state tradition limiting immunization mostly to the office of the private physician, no populationwide immunization programs had been implemented in Bowie County, Texas.

The Texarkana outbreak points up the excellence of measles as a sentinel disease. Measles is easily recognized

2. P. J. Landrigan, "Epidemic Measles in a Divided City," *Journal of the American Medical Association* 221 (August 7, 1972): pp. 567–570.

and is highly infectious. A known case will, on the average, transmit the disease to 85 percent of susceptible household contacts, and natural immunity occurs only as a result of having had the disease. All these facts add up to the conclusion that practically everyone in the population must be immunized if the spread of the disease is to be controlled. Moreover, after the first few months of life, every newborn baby is susceptible, so that there will always be a nonimmune population to test the efficacy of immunization programs.

If there had been an early warning system in operation in Texas in early 1970, a case of any one of these three sentinel diseases—diphtheria, poliomyelitis, or measles—could have alerted physicians or health authorities to the inadequacies of the state immunization program. If they were immediately rectified, unnecessary cases of measles, paralysis of some children by poliomyelitis, and deaths from diphtheria could have been prevented. In the same way, if there were an official list of sentinel health events and an operating branch in every medical care region, an early warning system could issue alerts, which, if heeded, could prevent much disease, disability, and untimely death in all parts of our country.

Converting the Numbers into Better Health 14

A guidance system and an early warning system integrated into a single functioning unit would provide the general data base and would serve as the heart of a national quality control system. The data would then be assayed in the light of accumulated scientific and technical knowledge in order to document the potential for health improvement and provide a solid basis for specific programs. There is a great need for a prestigious national agency, which I shall call the Federal Health Board, to encompass both of these functions and to perform the many other duties and responsibilities relevant to the scientific, professional, and technical documentation for constructive administrative policy, sound legislation, and realistic judicial decisions concerning medicine and medical care. The National Center for Health Statistics and the Center for Disease Control would become major entities within the Federal Health Board. If such a Board were created, it would become possible to effect the legislative, administrative, public, professional, scientific, and statistical action and collaboration needed to convert the numbers yielded by the quality control system into better health for all Americans.

The Federal Health Board

The creation of a prestigious Federal Health Board to act as a balance wheel for a national health program would fill an enormous gap. Advantage is not now taken of the body of accumulated medical knowledge and of the survey data of the National Center for Health Statistics or the epidemiological and laboratory data of the Center for Disease Control to obtain maximal health benefits from the expenditure of available funds.

Instead, governmental health decisions are taken individually as concessions are made to one or another political pressure. Witness the enactment of recent cancer legislation that is completely out of balance with efforts to control other diseases. Or consider the overly elaborate screening and medical care program for sickle cell anemia, a very serious illness which, unfortunately at the moment, can be prevented only by eugenic control, and for which treatment is symptomatic and promising research leads are few. Members of the Senate and the House who act as experts before Congressional committees testify on the toxicity of this or that drug or insecticide or on the cancer-producing effects of beef from cattle treated with estogenic hormones; and Monday morning quarterbacks without adequate scientific background or formal medical evaluation second-guess the ethics of medical research programs, the allocation of research funds by the National Institutes of Health, or activities of the Food and Drug Administration. Add to these politically generated pressures judicial decisions in which the admissibility of medical evidence depends more on the authority of the expert witness than on the scientific validity of the testimony. All such events occur because there is no agency in government with the prestige and authority to provide the scientific, professional, and technical knowledge, evaluation, and recommendations that are basic to constructive administrative policy and budgetary allocation, sound legislation, and realistic judicial decisions governing medical science and medical care.

To be sure, there have been heroic efforts, some very successful, by governmental agencies to produce sound, documented evaluations to meet emergencies particularly in the control of the communicable diseases. Thus, the tragedy of the deaths from Cutter vaccine at the time of the introduction of polio immunization led to the authoritative report from the Center for Disease Control upon which the production of safe Salk poliomyelitis vaccine is now based. The success of that effort established a precedent in government for objective evaluation that was followed in the decisions to substitute Sabin for Salk polio vaccine and to manufacture and distribute measles, rubella, and other vaccines. Over the years, the National Research Council affiliated with the National Academy of Sciences, the Office of Science and Technology in the Executive Department, and subunits of the Department of Health, Education, and Welfare, including the Center for Disease Control, and various of the

National Institutes of Health have produced authoritative statements that have guided governmental action. On the other hand, the National Institutes of Health have generally followed the policy that their primary mission is basic research and that they cannot be immediately responsible for the scientific content and validity of public health programs for the control of specific diseases. Thus, there is no systematic procedure for the production of documented, authoritative reports by governmental health agencies, and accomplishment has been spotty.

Furthermore, some agencies, even with the best of intentions, have not had adequate status to insist that scientific constraints be given their just consideration in political decisions. For example, the National Cancer Institute of the National Institutes of Health was not able to stand up to those administrators in the Office of the President who determined the final form of our misshapen cancer program. Indeed, the serious question was raised as to whether the national program on cancer should not be taken out of the National Institutes of Health and located within the White House. A compromise decision was reached in which the responsibility was divided. It is evident that scientific, professional, and technical constraints have not been taken adequately into account in many recent governmental health and medical care decisions.

But the converse is also true. Just as governmental officials should not make administrative, legislative, and judicial decisions concerning medicine and medical care without the basic scientific, professional, and technical input, so experts within or outside the proposed Federal Health Board should never make political or social governmental decisions by themselves. In a democracy, political decisions must be made by fully informed representatives of the people. The Federal Health Board should, however, supply the medical statesmanship to complement the political acumen that will be needed to institute and conduct a successful national health program. For clarification, let us accept a current definition of politics as "the art of the possible" and define statesmanship as the "science of the necessary." Obviously, both have to be carefully interwoven if scientific knowledge is to be translated into better human health.

There was no need for a federal health board when our country was founded in the late eighteenth century. Medical science was almost nonexistent and medical practice was rudimentary. But since that time, the doubling of the life expectancy and the improvement in the average level of health have expanded the lifetime opportunities of the individual and of society as a whole. The price of the scientific, professional, and technical medical progress in this century has been a congeries of unbelievable complexity and a continuing exponential rise in the cost of medical care, both of which have set off earthshaking social and political reverberations. Moreover, many special interest groups, including professional organizations, universities, hospitals, nursing home associations, insurance companies, industries, governmental agencies, political movements, labor unions, and consumers groups, have become involved, are operating independently, and in their eagerness to foster their own programs have confused the basic issues with their clouds of propaganda.

Medical care is now intricately intertwined with society, economics, and government. Moreover, the increasing complexity of many social problems has, in recent decades, engendered a growing public recognition of the need for government to participate in their resolution. We do need a preeminent, impartial institution to set the tone of, establish the guidelines for, and keep watch over the delivery of medical care. The new agency could guide the interweaving of the discoveries of medical science into an evolving program of medical care directed toward optimal individual and national health. The Federal Health Board would base its judgments on the facts of the situation as viewed against the tradition of clinical medicine, the body of scientific and technical knowledge, and the current status of national and regional health as revealed by the guidance system and the early warning system. If the Federal Health Board conducts this process of decision-making in a meticulous and thoughtful manner, it should soon acquire the prestige that will be essential to its effective operation.

Not an Administrative Agency

Before specifying the structure, membership, and the duties and responsibilities of the Federal Health Board, I want to be very specific about what the Board will not do. The Federal Health Board will not be the federal administrative agency for health and medical care. That responsibility will probably reside in the Department of Health, Education, and Welfare (see "Administration," chapter 17), depending, of course, on the final form of the national health program and other health legislation which will be enacted by the Congress. The best analogy in our national government for the relationship between the Federal Health Board and the administrative agency, the Department of Health, Education, and Welfare, is the relationship between the Federal Reserve Board and the Treasury Department. Just as the Federal Reserve Board is responsible for the control of credit, so would the Federal Health Board be responsible for the control of health. The Department of Health, Education, and Welfare, like the Department of the Treasury in financial matters, would continue to be the administrative arm of the Executive Department for health and medical care.

Structure and Membership

The Federal Health Board would be a quasi-independent agency consisting of nine members appointed for staggered long terms—about ten years, with possibility of reappointment until retirement at age 70—by the President with the approval of the Senate from a list of distinguished nominees submitted individually by each of a selected group of nongovernmental, prestigious, scientific medical organizations.[1] Since the Federal Health Board would be concerned solely with scientific, professional, and technical matters, each nominee should be a

1. Included in this group might be such organizations (listed alphabetically) as the American Academy of Arts and Sciences, American Academy of Pediatrics, American College of Physicians, American College of Surgeons, American Epidemiological Society, American Medical Association, American Society for Clinical Investigation, Association of American Medical Colleges, Association of American Physicians, The Institute of Medicine, and The National Academy of Sciences.

recognized authority in his field, and should have demonstrated the quality of statesmanship necessary to interrelate scientific and technical knowledge into governmental, political, and public endeavors for the improvement of health.

The membership of the Federal Health Board must be balanced among representatives of the major fields of knowledge related to medicine and medical care but it could not possibly provide representation for the many relevant disciplines, including all of the basic medical sciences and clinical specialties, and related areas such as engineering and economics. This is not to say that any one of these disciplines should not be included as long as the major criterion is the ability of the appointee to provide forward-looking guidance and leadership. Balanced representation of all relevant disciplines must, however, be assured through the membership of ad hoc expert committees that would be appointed by the Federal Health Board from all of the relevant disciplines to consider and to make recommendations concerning individual problems. Moreover, the full-time staff of the Federal Health Board, in addition to those of the National Center for Health Statistics and the Center for Disease Control, should include representation of many of the relevant disciplines, although part-time staff representing the more highly specialized ones would have to be appointed to meet specific needs. Whenever possible, for economy of cost and of personnel, for diversity and quality of advice, and to take advantage of existing institutions—the universities, the National Academy of Sciences, and the Institute of Medicine—the

Federal Health Board should draw heavily on outside advisors and advisory institutions and not build up a huge, isolated, in-house professional staff.

Regional Health Boards
In parallel with the Federal Health Board at the national level, there would be established in each medical care region an affiliated regional health board. (For the method of appointment of the regional health board and its interaction with state governments, see "Local Health Administration," chapter 17.) Each regional health board using the data of the quality control system would be responsible for the assay of and recommendations for the improvement of health in its region. The Federal Health Board would provide each regional health board with analyses of the health of its region compared with that of other regions and the nation as a whole. The Federal Health Board would also call attention to preventable and remediable conditions that impair the health of each region. In turn, each regional health board would report on its activities and its successes and failures in the improvement of regional health. It would also advise the Federal Health Board on specific improvements and changes needed in the operation of the quality control system. In a word, the regional health boards would act as the agents of the Federal Health Board to assay health and to guide medical care at the regional level.

Medical care regions centering on medical school affiliated hospitals would be more efficient if they were congruent with local marketing areas and took advantage of established communication and transportation systems. As was pointed out earlier, many existing medical service areas obviously cross state lines; western Massachusetts, for example, centers on Albany Medical College in Albany, New York, and southeastern Massachusetts on Brown University in Providence, Rhode Island. As is true of the credit control activities of the Federal Reserve Board, the quality control program of the Federal Health Board would eliminate the artificial barrier of state lines that cut across and divide medical service areas. The direct affiliation of each regional health board with the Federal Health Board will preserve efficient local medical service areas and will be flexible enough to adjust to the evolution of new service areas as local industries and occupations shift and change with the times.

Duties of the Federal Health Board

The Federal Health Board would have many vital duties and responsibilities. It would:
1. guide the planning and implementation of the conversion of existing resources into a single national health program;
2. continuously assay the state of and pinpoint measures to improve national and regional health;
3. use established indices and when appropriate create new indices of health to identify preventable and remediable causes of unnecessary disease, disability, and untimely death;
4. document scientific, professional, and technical evalu-

ations that are essential and basic to constructive administrative policy in the Executive Department, sound legislation by the Congress, and realistic decisions by the Judiciary relevant to medicine, medical care, and the health of the American people;
5. recommend priorities for the expenditure of the national health budget to attain the highest possible levels of health;
6. identify national health emergencies and local health emergency areas;
7. develop and maintain within the structure of Congressional legislation, a national health code governing such matters as standards of programs of care and of environmental health, and qualifications of professional and allied professional personnel; and
8. establish closely knit liaison with the Congressional Office of Health Care (chapter 15) to give adequate and thorough consideration to interests and needs of purveyors and consumers of medical care prior to final decisions concerning scientific, professional, and technical health matters, and to aid in consumer education.

1. **Guide the Conversion into the National Health Program.**

The key question in the organization of a national health program to provide optimal care is, How can the present chaotic nonsystem be converted into a single program that will use existing resources to the maximum extent and yet preserve the freedom to explore and the spirit of originality so essential to its continuing constructive evolution? There will be many answers to this question at both national and regional levels, depending upon the phase of program integration, the quality of existing resources, and the political climate. The answers cannot be anticipated. Instead, they must be arrived at after careful study by an agency with great prestige, research competence, practical expertise, and the ability to obtain public support.

I believe that the proposed Federal Health Board with the collaborative assistance of the Congressional Office of Health Care would meet the criteria and its members would have the qualifications to accomplish the delicate process of conversion. It could also aid the administrative agency, the Department of Health, Education, and Welfare, in the implementation of an operating program. The membership of the Federal Health Board, having been selected in its very special way, would consist of outstanding leaders in medicine and in health and medical care delivery. Another great asset of the Federal Health Board is its responsibility for quality control, incorporating within its structure the administrative units concerned with the collection and analysis of the data in the guidance system and early warning system. The membership of the ad hoc committees of the Federal Health Board would include representatives of all the disciplines relevant to the solution of crucial problems in the planning and evolution of the national health program. The staff of the Federal Health Board would have the background and competence to crystallize the recommendations of the Board into the form needed by the administrative agency to carry out its program. Finally, the close working relationship with the Congressional Office of Health Care throughout this whole process of conversion would take into account the needs of the public and would obtain the necessary public support for the administrative agency in the implementation of the program.

Let us examine the process of conversion and use emergency care, the first step in the evolution of the total program, as an example. An optimal regional emergency care plan would be developed by the Department of Health, Education, and Welfare under the guidance of the Federal Health Board in cooperation with the Congressional Office of Health Care. At the local level, the regional health board would examine, evaluate, and classify local resources that might fit or be modified to fit the national plan of conversion as adapted to meet local needs. The next step in conversion would be the identification of lacks in hospital, communication, transportation, and personnel requirements, and the development of a program to close the gaps in the most effective and economical way. During the process, as individual modules are converted or created they would be tested by actual experience in the field. To facilitate this process of conversion throughout the country, experience gained in individual areas would be integrated into the national planning process by the Federal Health Board and channeled in an educational program to all the health regions of the country.

In this blueprint the order of procedure in creating individual modules begins with regional health organization, goes on to emergency care, and then to ambulatory care, first tied into inpatient services and finally into a total regional program. But actual timing in any one region will depend upon available resources, the opportunity for the adaptation of old and the creation of new entities, and the best timing of their integration. Moreover, if a national health program is to become a reality, it is essential that in the very earliest stages of legislation for the national program provision must be made for the establishment of the Federal Health Board, the regional health boards, a Congressional Office of Health Care, and the administrative expansion in the Department of Health, Education, and Welfare.

One essential point: the integration of an existing institution or agency into a national health program must preserve the spirit of independence and originality so necessary for continuous constructive improvement of medical care. We must continue the kind of environment in our great teaching hospitals that has been mainly responsible for the evolution of valuable superspecialist services such as the surgery of kidney transplantation. Research workers must have the opportunity to explore, initiate, and try out life-saving procedures. Also, the pioneering prepayment group practice organizations must continue to have the freedom and the scope to try out new methods of health care delivery. The Federal Health Board, under the stimulus of the quality control system, would maintain throughout the entire health care system the atmosphere of academic freedom that is so essential to basic and applied medical and medical care research and to constantly improving performance. That accomplishment alone would obstruct the development of a stultifying bureaucracy. There is an excellent precedent in the National Health Service of the United

Kingdom. Those who planned that Service had the foresight to set aside, in accounts separate from the general budget, the endownments and research funds of the medical school teaching hospitals for research expenditure under conditions as free as those now in effect in the United States. Likewise in the United States, research budgets have been kept separate from the funds allocated for medical care in the intramural and extramural programs of the National Institutes of Health and such institutions as the Health Research Institute of the City of New York.

Detailed planning and integration of the national health program and the maintenance of its vitality will be the most difficult task of all. Under the relentless pressure of controlling the costs of health and medical care services, the Federal Health Board, acting together with the Congressional Office of Health Care and the Department of Health, Education, and Welfare, should be able to effect the conversion of the existing situation into a single, continually improving national health program.

2. Assay National and Regional Health, and Pinpoint Measures for Improvement

The Federal Health Board, by means of the quality control program of its constituent agencies, the National Center for Health Statistics and the Center for Disease Control, would keep continuous watch over the state of national and regional health. The Board would then compare actual health status with the potential level of health that could be reached by optimal use of the accumulated body of medical knowledge. Deficits would be identified that would become the focal points for optimal health improvement. In actual practice, the optimal program would then have to be scaled down to fit into the existing and potential range of medical, economic, institutional, personnel, and social resources. The Federal Health Board would, of course, have the constant responsibility to increase such resources to a maximum and to recommend their fair allotment among all of the health regions of the country.

But resources will always lag behind needs. To guide the scaling down process from optimal to actual objectives, the Federal Health Board will have to establish and maintain a current list of priorities based on the relative importance of the gaps in health services and the feasibility of their eradication. In this process, advantage should be taken of systems analysis and operations research to identify the linkages and trade-offs necessary to reach the highest possible level of national and regional health within the limitations of available and potential resources. As a result of all these efforts, specific recommendations would be made to each agency responsible for the administration of the national health program and its regional affiliates. In a word, the Federal Health Board would guide the application of the finite medical, economic, institutional, personnel, and social resources to elevate health status as closely as possible to theoretically optimal levels.

3. **Establish New Indices of Health**

Because the health picture is constantly changing, the Federal Health Board will have to reevaluate its methods of health assay constantly in order to define the status of major health problems and to take aim with riflelike precision at the individual elements of preventable and treatable causes of unnecessary disease, disability, and untimely death. Diseases do wax and wane in their human virulence. In our lifetime, scarlet fever has lost its fatal bite, while in the overnourished countries, coronary heart disease has assumed epidemic proportions. An alert watch will have to be kept to be sure that the samples, methods, interview questions, physical examinations, and laboratory procedures used in the guidance system remain relevant to national and regional health, and that the list of sentinel diseases in the early warning system remains up to date. Within the constraints imposed by the need for following carefully defined health trends over time, every effort must be made to concentrate on the collection of those data that most clearly pinpoint remediable gaps in medical care so as to effect immediate improvement in the health of the population.

With such information and to accomplish its ends, the Federal Health Board will establish and maintain a set of sensitive and relevant indices of health to guide the national health program and indicate to the population at large the current status of national and regional health. Thus, in the guidance system with the resources of the National Center for Health Statistics, it should be possible to develop and maintain a series of quantitative indices, each of which would indicate the status of an important health problem and/or the effectiveness of the control of a remediable cause of ill health. Similarly, in the early warning system, with resources of the Center for Disease Control, the indices could be presented as a box score of successes and failures in the prevention and control of those sentinel events of ill health that should occur rarely or take place only within specified limits in any country or region with an up-to-date health and medical care program. As time goes on, individual indices may have to be discarded, created, or modified if we are to be constantly informed as to the status of major problems, identify remediable gaps in health care, and be aware of the actual level of control of preventable and treatable threats to life and health.

4. Document Scientific, Professional, and Technical Evaluations of Medicine, Medical Care, and Health

The Federal Health Board would become the recognized source of thoroughly documented evaluations of the nation's health and of the state of scientific knowledge, professional capability, and technology relevant to the solution of specific important current health problems.

The Federal Health Board would prepare statements of evaluation in response to many different kinds of stimuli, some inherent in the quality control system, and others upon request of another governmental agency. The quality control system might reveal, for example, a sudden increase in the death rate from exposure to asbestos. The march of medical progress might uncover the need for a precise evaluation of intensive care units in the treatment of heart attacks. The Executive Department might request a statement to serve as the scientific basis for a policy to maintain adequate nutrition of infants and small children during a food shortage. The Congress, considering narcotic legislation, might require scientific testimony on the value of methadone or whatever other treatment is being recommended for control of heroin addiction. The Supreme Court might, for its guidance, need a carefully balanced, documented opinion of the specific danger of a particular environmental health hazard, for example, automobile exhaust emissions.

Objective scientific, professional, and technical evaluation would become the hallmark of the Federal Health Board and would provide a sound basis for its prestige and its authority. Often, there will not be enough knowledge extant to document a definitive evaluation. For example, if the Federal Health Board were requested to provide an evaluation of acupuncture, it would make a tentative report and the uncertain nature of the evaluation would be clearly stated. Most important, the preliminary appraisal of the Board would specify the state of relevant knowledge and the kinds of controlled studies and epidemiologic observations needed to collect the information essential to definitive evaluation. In the event of disagreement within the Board, both majority and minority opinions would be made public. Most important of all, in every statement of evaluation the Federal Health Board would make crystal clear which decisions are based on solid facts, that is, reproducible observations, and which decisions are judgmental. It would specify whatever additional knowledge might be needed to place the scientific, professional, or technical evaluation on an objective basis. Such practice is essential to the guidance of a sound national health program and would give the public a better understanding of how scientific knowledge derived from research is essential to their health. It should also increase their confidence in the efforts to apply scientific knowledge in the prevention and the treatment of their diseases.

5. Recommend Priorities in Expenditure of the National Health Budget to Attain Highest Possible Levels of Health

To convert the numbers into better health, there must be a direct feedback from the quality control system to the budgetary allocation of funds among the many facets of the health and medical care program. To be sure, the Executive Department through the Secretary of Health, Education, and Welfare and the Office of Management and Budget, after having taken into consideration the documented recommendations of the Federal Health Board concerning total health needs, will establish the resource priorities between health and other fields. With its distinguished membership, the Federal Health Board will have the qualifications both to balance the evidence of unfulfilled needs, the potential application of the body of medical knowledge within the constraints of medical, economic, institutional, personnel, and social resources, and the accomplishments and failures of existing health programs, and also to use such integrated information to recommend priorities to the Department of Health, Education, and Welfare, to the Office of Management and Budget, and to the Congress concerning the distribution of the economic resources allocated for health and medical care. To perform this complex task, the Federal Health Board must have the specific authority in its enabling legislation that assigns to it the key *advisory* role in the distribution of available funds among the various health and medical care needs. For practical implementation of its responsibilities, the staff of the Board must work closely with the staffs of Congressional committees and representatives of the Secretary of the Department of Health, Education, and Welfare, Congressional Office of Health Care, Office of Management and Budget, and other agencies, such as the Veterans' Administration, which are also concerned with the provision of medical care. There would be one major exception. Although the Federal Health Board would make general recommendations concerning the areas where medical research expenditures should be concentrated, it would leave to the National Institutes of Health and their advisory councils and expert committees their present responsibility for making individual recommendations in the allocation of research funds to research institutions and to investigators.

In government, an agency whose authority is advisory is not likely to exert much influence on the expenditure of funds. If the role of the Federal Health Board were merely that of an isolated body producing reports, it would accomplish little in the improvement of the nation's health. But in its proposed key role in the assay of health, and with its complex task, as herein defined, the Federal Health Board should be in the best position to make clear to the government and to the public the reasons for specific budgetary allocations of health and medical care funds. If its membership is properly chosen and it performs its task well, the Federal Health Board will develop the prestige to give it great influence in the allocation of funds for individual facets of health and medical care. In any event, precise wording in the enabling legislation must make clear the complex role of the Federal Health Board and its responsibility for translating the numbers measuring the quality of medical care into better health for Americans.

6. Identify National Health Emergencies and Local Health Emergency Areas

The Federal Health Board should be given the authority to identify and recommend to the President the designation of national health emergencies and local health emergency areas. The recommendations would include the scientific, professional, and technical documentation to support the designation and the procedures to be followed in meeting the emergency. This process would be parallel to the existing practice of designation of disaster areas by the President of the United States.

7. Develop a National Health Code

The manifold activities of the Federal Health Board will demand that the scientific, professional, and technical standards, criteria, and recommendations that relate to health programs be classified in some orderly fashion and be implemented in accordance with a defined procedure. To meet this need, it is recommended that there be established, within the framework of federal law, a national health code consisting of regulations enacted by the Federal Health Board and concerned with the application of scientific, professional, and technological standards and criteria in the design and operation of public health and medical care programs. In effect the code based on the body of medical knowledge and the needs revealed by the quality control system, would lay down the guidelines for the organization of specific programs, such as an emergency care transportation system or a communication system for consultation at a distance, to keep unnecessary disease, disability, and untimely death at minimal levels.

The code would not, like that of the Internal Revenue Service, prescribe all the fine details of and act like a straightjacket on every local health program. Instead, it would supply general guidelines and would be supplemented by a proposed regional health code that could be modified by each regional health board to meet local needs. The national health code would be changed in response to new medical knowledge and to information yielded by the quality control system. But it should be clear that the effectiveness of national and regional health programs would be determined by the quality control system and not by compliance with the national health code.

The national health code could have many direct and indirect beneficial applications. At the national level, by fitting together in its regulations the existing body of medical knowledge and the current status of health as revealed by the quality of control system, the code could guide the more effective budgeting of funds for medical care. At the regional level, it could serve as a navigational chart in laying out a course toward better health. The code could also be the basis for a better understanding between the public and the medical professions and help do away with quackery. Thus, the requirements of the code would suggest to the public what benefits it could reasonably expect from modern medical care and would protect the physician against unwarranted malpractice suits. In a word, just as the quality control system is the measuring stick for the state of health of the population, so will the national health code become the fixed reference point for the procedures to be instituted for the improvement of health.

8. Establish Liaison with the Congressional Office of Health Care

In this blueprint, the decisions, priorities, and recommendations concerning consumer needs and responsibilities are allocated to the Office of Health Care to be created in the Congress to represent the public interest. The duties and responsibilities of the Congressional Office of Health Care with membership from both Houses are, thus, distinctly different from the purely scientific, professional, and technical ones that require the specialized competence of members of the Federal Health Board. This Office should be given the opportunity, except in acute emergencies, to review recommendations of the Federal Health Board to be sure that the public interest is taken adequately into account in their implementation. In turn and in the same way, the Federal Health Board should have the opportunity to review the recommendations of the Congressional Office of Health Care to be sure that they are consistent with the scientific, professional, and technical considerations that govern delivery of efficient, high quality medical care. Such interactive liaison should facilitate the improvement of and remove obstructions to the operation of national and regional health programs.

In actual practice, to insure effective operation, the members and staffs of the Federal Health Board and the Congressional Office of Health Care would keep each other currently informed on matters of mutual interest and make every effort to iron out potential disagreements prior to final recommendations by either agency. Liaison must be very efficient and bureaucratic wrangling must be avoided so that precious time is not wasted in bringing health benefits to the people. It may be anticipated that sound scientific, professional, and technical recommendations will at times introduce hardships for the health professions or for the public, or may appear to introduce hurdles in the improvement of health. On the other hand, comsumer or purveyor recommendations may be in conflict with the import of existing scientific knowledge, be beyond professional competence, or be technically unfeasible. In resolving all such disagreements, highest priority must always be given to the health of the people. In the event of truly insoluble differences, each agency must be free to submit its recommendations together with any minority reports to the Executive Department and to the Congress. It is also essential that controversial recommendations be publicized in order to arrive at statesmanlike and politically feasible solutions to serious health problems at the earliest possible moment.

The quality control system under the supervision of a prestigious Federal Health Board and as advised by the Congressional Office of Health Care, is the keystone of the edifice of the medicine of the future portrayed in this blueprint. Its creation need not wait upon the establishment of a national health program. Much research will be needed to modify the data collection of the National Center for Health Statistics in its various surveys, to interweave the surveillance functions of the Center for Disease Control, and to forge and validate a precise instrument which would focus on unnecessary undesirable health events so that they might be eliminated. The Center for Disease Control would develop a new focus of interest by making on-the-spot investigations of outcroppings of unnecessary disease, disability, or untimely death. Indeed, as indicated in chapter 13, the Center for Disease Control, in cooperation with the National Center for Health Statistics would direct the early warning system. In this grave moment in the history of health services in the United States, with the rapid turnover of personnel at the highest level in an unstable national health administration, we sorely need a quality control system to monitor the state of our national health, to document the need for an effective national health administration, and to guide us in the design and operation of a national health program for the improvement of our national health and for the prevention and treatment of disease. We must create a quality control system now!

The Public Interest 15

The main objectives of a national health program are the maintenance of health and the effective prevention and treatment of the illnesses of all of the people. These objectives are constantly obscured by the many issues raised by special interest groups justifiably concerned about their future roles and rewards when a national health program goes into operation. To be sure, every effort must be made to satisfy the needs and desires of all those concerned with the provision of medical care.

But the public interest must be primary. That interest will best be served by the provision of high quality medical care in a manner that conveniently and effectively brings together the program and the people. The maintenance of efficient high quality medical care will be the responsibility of the Federal Health Board and its affiliated regional health boards. The blueprint must, therefore, propose a mechanism whereby high quality medical care is made available to the people in the most convenient way. For each individual, the patient's own physician will serve as the channel of communication. But there must also be liaison at the national, regional, and district levels so that the public interest is taken into account in establishing policy, planning the national health program, budgeting funds, and instituting new medical care procedures, as well as in keeping the public informed about the most effective ways in which to use the medical care system.

At the National Level

At the national level, a channel must be created by which the administration is kept informed of the public interest so that it may be given adequate consideration in the planning and operation of the program. The usual vehicle is a committee of outstanding citizens appointed by the President with the approval of the Senate or by the administrator of the program. But it is almost impossible to be sure that an appointed national committee will really represent the public. There are so many special interest groups concerned with medical care. Moreover, prominent citizens are loath to accept a long-term, continuous commitment that may keep them occupied almost full time.

The Congressional Office of Health Care could serve this watchdog function admirably. It would take an active part in the planning of the national health program and would constantly survey and evaluate its public effect. The Congress is the most appropriate body because its members are elected and it comes closest to representing the public interest. There is a precedent in the recent establishment of the Office of Technology Assessment by the Congress. Moreover, in the past, watchdog committees of the Congress—the Truman Senate Special Committee Investigating the National Defense Program during World War II, among others—have performed distinguished service. As needed, the Congressional Office of Health Care would appoint temporary committees of distinguished citizens to investigate, study, and report to the Congress on the state of the public's interest in individual, urgent public health and medical care problems, such as public policy on the provision of artificial kidney dialysis. The public interest would also be furthered by open hearings at stated times where prominent and concerned citizens could testify on major nontechnical health issues such as public policy on contraception and abortion. Thus, the Congressional Office would have a double function: the assessment of factors affecting the public interest and a channel whereby public opinion could make itself known and felt.

This proposal will be objected to on the grounds that because of its extensive legislative commitments, the Congress cannot establish a watchdog committee for every important national program. It will also be pointed out that its heterogeneous membership and its almost nonexistent central administrative structure prevent the Congress from operating as a single unit. But these are exactly the reasons why the Congress is now in such great difficulty in implementing its legislative intentions through programs administered by the Executive Department. If it is to have equal influence in our system of checks and balances, the Congress must have a central administrative structure strong enough to assure that its legislative intentions are implemented by the programs of the Executive Department. As heterogeneous as the Congress is, it does agree on major issues by majority vote and does enact legislation. Moreover, the large proportion of gross national product—8.3 percent, equivalent to more than eighty billion dollars—spent on health is of major concern to the Congress. A national health program to improve the health of the entire public might be a very good place for the Congress to start in the development of its central administration to redress the serious imbalance in our national government.

The Congressional Office of Health Care could make its influence felt in many ways. Within the Congress, representatives of the Congressional Office of Health Care would testify and report their findings before the appropriations committees, the Senate Finance Committee, and the House Committee on Ways and Means. Each Congressman would serve as a conduit between his constituents and the Congressional Office of Health Care. Most important, the findings of the Congressional Office of Health Care would be interwoven with those on the quality and efficiency of medical care of the Federal Health Board and transmitted to the regional health boards for planning of local medical care services and in recommending priorities in the budgeting of funds for the local programs. If this system were made operative, the public interest would be well served.

At the Local Level
At the district level (figure 3), where medical care is actively practiced, the public interest is directly involved.

The district medical care program, in addition to guiding each individual to medical care, must provide for the expression and implementation of the public's interest, educate the public in the effective use of the program, inform the entire staff of the needs of the public so that these will be taken fully into account in the planning and provision of medical services, and alert those patients who need help and could benefit from immediate care.

Every reception center in every medical care district (figure 3) should provide channels of communication between the community, the purveyors of medical care, and the administrators of the program. The channels would permit the exchange of information on such matters as the elimination of inadequacies, for example, irregular night transportation, the improvement of services through, say, a more efficient appointment system, and specific complaints about the management of individual patients. The major channel would be a citizens' committee to represent the people of the district. In order that the district reception center be the focal point, space within it should be provided where at stated meetings of the citizens' committee and of other local groups information would be exchanged and recommendations made concerning the solution of specific problems.

The Education Program

Education at the local level in the use of a new system of medical care must reach two groups: the beneficiaries of services and the providers of care. The beneficiaries must be well informed so that they may take full advantage of available resources. The providers of care must be cognizant of the needs of the population and of the relative effectiveness of each of the elements of the program. In a sense, education must become the lubricant of the interaction between the centrifugal flow of scientific and professional knowledge and services from the central and community hospitals and the district reception centers and the centripetal streams of defined medical care needs from the people living in the districts served by the program. All will be guided in their quest for better health if the educational curricula include pertinent data and the recommendations of the quality control system. The gaps in local health services that must be repaired will be identified by the regional health board by comparing the actual state of health in the local area with the standards of optimal attainable health of the quality control system. Optimal attainable health is the best that can be expected from the effective implementation of existing scientific, professional, and technical knowledge. The actual status of health would be determined by the level of unnecessary disease, disability, and untimely death determined by the guidance system and the early warning system, supplemented by whatever other evidence exists of locally uncontrolled but manageable health problems.

Confidence is essential to community acceptance of new patterns of medical care. American patients able to afford a physician and needing medical care are accustomed to depending upon him alone as if he were able all by himself or with the assistance of consultants to provide all aspects of care. The patient unable to pay for care or to find a private doctor expects to be greeted by a white-suited physician in the hospital outpatient department, in the emergency room, or in the isolated community health center. Medical consumers of the system proposed by this blueprint will discover that the new variety of ambulatory care is better than the mere availability of a physician. They will understand why a solo practitioner cannot provide modern scientific medicine alone and why he needs the support of professional and technological personnel and the assistance of modern medical machinery. They must agree that the time of the physician has to be reserved for those tasks that only he can perform and that are essential to the patient's care. They must not demand that a physician provide them with services that can be supplied as effectively by specially trained allied health personnel. Each medical consumer must adjust to the idea that he will make his first contact with the triage nurse, who with the assistance of other allied health personnel, will provide minor care, encouragement, and reassurance and will refer the patient forthwith to his personal physician whenever he is really needed. This proposed triage plan is far better than the present haphazard arrangement. Now it us usually the office nurse or secretary untrained in triage who, with or without the intervention of an answering service, decides if and when the patient will see his physician. Finally, if they are to derive maximum benefits from the proposed program, it is essential that the people should learn that they must participate actively in the educational process.

Education of the Staff

Similarly, on their part, the professional, administrative, technical, and service staff must be kept currently aware of their respective roles in the total program, the changing patterns of local needs, the degree to which the needs are being met, and the specific unmet needs that could be satisfied by program readjustment. They will learn from the quality control system the details of both their successes and their failures in suppressing unnecessary disease, disability, and untimely death in the most efficient way. Indeed, they must always measure their accomplishments against the established professional standards and health indices of the quality control system and be willing to make appropriate changes whenever clearly indicated. Finally, the staff must understand the reasons for and the details of recommended remedial measures so that they may be adjusted to local conditions and be accomplished within the limitations of the established priority list and with the most efficient use of available funds and personnel.

The Health Alerting System

In the final analysis, acceptance of a new medical care program will depend upon the actual demonstration that high quality medical care is available when needed. Moreover, if prevention and early treatment are to do the most good, care cannot wait until the average individual realizes that he is in trouble. Instead, his needs must be anticipated. This fact has been recognized in maternal and infant care, in immunization against serious illness such as diphtheria and poliomyelitis, and in screening programs for early cancer detection such as that of the uterine cervix. But these are preventive programs for the entire community or for special risk groups. They are not designed to meet the day-by-day needs of an individual who has a special medical problem. In this blueprint, through the proposed health alerting system, it would become possible for the first time to anticipate individual medical care needs and to arrange for immediate referral to appropriate medical care.

Individual preventive and early treatment services are delicate to arrange because one may properly raise the issue of violation of the privacy of the person who does not wish to have such services. In a democratic society, the reasons for a particular preventive or therapeutic procedure must be clearly stated so that everyone may have the available facts when he makes his own decision on the acceptance of care. But the decision is his alone, as long as his refusal does not threaten the health of others. The proposed health alerting system must, therefore, always be permissive, never compulsive.

There are many easily identifiable events to indicate that available preventive or therapeutic medical care resources could be helpful to the individual who does not know that he needs help. The record of a marriage, a birth, a hospital admission, a serious accident, a laboratory report "positive" for a communicable disease, pregnancy, cancer, or high blood cholesterol are all examples of easily identifiable events that could trigger the health alerting system to determine whether full advantage is being taken of the health care program, whether medical care should be initiated, or whether all available resources are being efficiently used. All such triggering events are already being recorded somewhere in the community but their existence is often ignored and their use in improving the health and medical care of each person is irregularly applied by public health and medical care agencies.

It remains for the health officer-hospital administrator in the proposed blueprint, with his office in the hospital rather than in city hall, to identify all available items of information that could serve to alert patients to the need for medical care. He must systematically examine all sorts of health data available anywhere in the community and ask the question, Could the use of this item of health information act as a trigger in a health alerting system? If the answer is Yes, provision must be made for the collection of that particular item on a continuing basis and for its use in the health-alerting system.

A mechanism must be established so that when a positive report is made and if available resources are not being used, and if the person will accept assistance, a telephone call or, when necessary, a home visit by a public health nurse would provide an entry point to care. The nurse's visit in time of need would aid in cementing relationships with the reception center staff and in building the confidence of the community in the medical care program. It should also demonstrate to the individual the personal interest of those responsible for his care. But it must be remembered that the visit by itself is a mechanism and not the objective. The important step is the actual satisfaction of individual medical care needs, including assurance that the patient's personal physician will be accessible when his services are required. The final objective will be the high quality of medical care actually provided as indicated by the state of health of the local population determined by the quality control system.

As the health alerting system is established, its operation would be integrated with the general preventive and the screening programs on the one hand and the emergency medical service on the other. In the first instance, it would urge immediate therapeutic services for those in the beginning stages of diseases that are better treated early than late. Next, it would call attention to the need for preventive services for people at high risk, such as heart-attack-prone individuals who have high blood pressure or high blood cholesterol or are heavy cigarette smokers. And if prevention fails and the heart attack does occur, appropriate liaison with the emergency medical care service could assist in bringing very early treatment to the patient when it might make the difference between life and death.

Thus, at national, regional, and district levels and in many ways, the public must learn how to use the health care system, and, in turn, the public interest must be taken into account in establishing policies on the operation of the system and the ways in which care is given to each individual.

Payment to the Physician 16

The practice of medicine places severe demands on the physician. After a long and expensive period of education and training, he plays the decisive role in the maintenance of health and in the prevention and treatment of disease. Whenever the presence of the patient's physician can make a real difference in the outcome or management of a life-threatening or other major illness, he should be available himself or should arrange for a competent substitute who knows enough about the patient and his illness to provide adequate care.

The implications are clear. A physician cannot practice good medicine within the constraints of a forty-hour week. Although he must have ample time off from practice for rest and relaxation and for his family, in order to practice good medicine he will at times have to place the welfare of his patient above his personal needs and desires. If the physician accepts such responsibility, he should be well paid for his efforts and should be given incentive payments for exceptional accomplishments and for extraordinary sacrifices, to motive him to bring better medical care to his patients.

In the United States, the physician is compensated through a fee-for-service system in which he bills the patient, the insurance company, or the government for each individual service provided to the patient. Regardless of the development of a national health program, the fee-for-service method of payment will continue for those who prefer to obtain their medical care on a private basis. This is true in countries that already have well-functioning national health and medical care programs, such as Sweden and the United Kingdom.

The fee-for-service system does have the serious limitation that the total cost of physician services over any period of time is unpredictable. Moreover, the open-ended arrangement whereby the physician himself determines the kind and number of procedures for which he will then be remunerated may be a motivating factor in overtreatment. Indeed, there is much evidence that the number of elective surgical procedures is correlated with the patient's ability to pay.

The fee-for-service system of payment has tended to hold back the evolution of prepayment insurance for total medical care. When the total cost of professional services cannot be budgeted, it becomes impossible to predict the size of the premium that will insure for the total cost of care. To control total professional care costs, as in Medicare and Medicaid, and in Blue Cross-Blue Shield and private insurance contracts, all kinds of deductibles, exclusions, and limitations are introduced, with the result that medical care tends to be incomplete, fiscal accounting becomes infinitely complex, and administration is very expensive. Now that the need for total medical care is becoming more and more apparent and the cost of medical care continues its exponential growth, there are increasing demands for fixed and predictable budgets to cover complete medical care for everyone.

A modified fee-for-service system with built-in controls has been attempted in Sweden. Until recently when a salaried payment system was introduced, the patient would pay the physician's fee and then would be reimbursed a fixed amount by the Swedish government for each physician's service. This gave the patient a strong incentive to keep the physician's fee from being far in excess of the fixed reimbursement. There is no such motivation in the fee-for-service system in the United States, where the government or the insurance company pays the fee directly to the physician. However, it is not clear from the record nor from my conversations with officials of the Swedish Health Board whether the patient was actually able to control the size of his physician's fee or why the method of payment was given up.

Proposed Method of Payment

To meet the needs of physicians and a national medical care program, the following method of payment is recommended. Each general physician and specialist would be paid a salary supplemented by incentive awards. The salary should be generous enough to attract new members to the profession and to compensate for the costs of, and lack of income during, the prolonged period of education. It should also be adjusted to the specialty of the physician to assure an adequate number of each kind of specialist. Moreover, it is imperative that the general physician be compensated in the same range as the specialist in order to influence medical students to become general physicians.

As supplements to the physician's salary, incentive awards should be granted to the physician by the regional health board with the approval of the Federal Health Board for:
1. special contributions to medical knowledge and to medical care;
2. unusual hazards or hardships in his service; and,
3. most important of all, to motivate him to bring better medical care to his patients.

The physician may be granted incentive awards repeatedly whenever his accomplishments justify them. Once granted, the incentive award would become a permanent addition to his salary.

Incentive awards for meritorious contributions by specialists have been granted in the United Kingdom for many years and have apparently worked well for both the public and the profession. However, they have not been successful for British general practitioners because of the difficulty of identifying their relative contributions to medical care. In this blueprint, it is recommended that whenever they can be precisely determined, unusual and meritorious contributions by the physician to medicine and medical care be rewarded by incentive payments.

Physicians should be given incentive payments to practice in remote areas or under hazardous conditions.

The regional system of medical care, with the teaching hospital affiliated with the medical school as the focal point, should in great measure increase the attractiveness of medical practice even in relatively remote areas. Nevertheless, in our increasingly urbanized society, it will be essential that the attractiveness of such practice be enhanced by incentive payments.

The effective practice of high-quality medical care in a region provides an additional, and perhaps the most important, basis for making incentive awards to general physicians and to specialists. The crucial index is the infrequency of those varieties of unnecessary disease, disability, and untimely death that are clearly the direct responsibility of the physician. The index would also take seriously into account those instances of unnecessary disease, disability, and untimely death that are actually created by the doctor, for example, those due to unnecessary surgery or to the improper use of drugs.

There is evidence that incentive awards do influence the way the physician practices his profession. Physicians in the Kaiser-Permanente Program, whose financial incentive award system is designed to shift patients from the inpatient to ambulatory care facilities, have decreased the demand for hospital beds by the performance of an increasing proportion of their diagnostic workups on ambulatory patients. I believe that physicians could be motivated to practice more preventive medicine and to provide more effective therapeutic care if the resulting decrease in unnecessary disease, disability, or untimely death were recognized by granting financial incentive awards. At first, the measurements of quality and the

Proposed Method of Payment 241

incentive payments to doctors will have to be regionwide. Eventually, when the quality control system is working effectively, it could be used to identify specific hospitals and individual physicians in the region that deserve financial recognition for having improved the quality of medical care for their patients. In a word, physicians will get paid more if they keep their patients well.

Whatever the basis for the payment of physicians in our future national health service, two things must be clear: the total professional care costs must be predictable in an annual budget; and the unusual demands that the practice of medicine places on the conscientious physician must be compensated for by generous financial rewards.

Administration

17

It is assumed that the Department of Health, Education, and Welfare will be responsible for the administration of whatever national health program is enacted by the Congress. This assumption is, of course, subject to congressional legislation that may carve a Department of Health out of the Department of Health, Education, and Welfare or may allocate responsibility for a national health program to another agency. These recommendations on administration and financing of a national health program would be applicable in any of these situations.

A Historical Note
Recent catastrophic developments in our national health administration make it necessary to review its history. The success of the proposed national health program will depend upon an efficient administrative structure in which the political, and the scientific, professional ele-

A Historical Note

ments are carefully defined, separated, and then placed in proper balance with each other.

The administrative responsibility for the health of the nation has been ambiguous since the creation of the Department of Health, Education, and Welfare in 1952. That reorganization did transfer into the Department from the Federal Security Agency many of the administrative units concerned with health services, including the United States Public Health Service, the Children's Bureau, the Food and Drug Administration, and the Office of Vocational Rehabilitation. The chain of command at the very top was complicated by the creation, at the urging of the American Medical Association, of a new political officer—first called an Assistant to the Secretary of Health, Education, and Welfare—whose policy-making responsibilities threatened to overlap those of the Surgeon General of the United States Public Health Service, the top career officer in the major administrative agency for health. In spite of the lack of precise definition of administrative responsibility, the system worked quite well because (1) by law, certain clearly defined responsibilities were assigned to the Surgeon General of the United States Public Health Service; (2) the Public Health Service was a large nationwide service organization while the Office of the Assistant Secretary comprised a tiny, limited group of administrators; and (3) the incumbents of the Office of the Assistant Secretary were, for the most part, highly competent, responsible, cooperative individuals who did their best to foster the total program.

The reallocation of professional and scientific responsibilities from career officers to political appointees began with the reorganization of the Department of Health, Education, and Welfare by Undersecretary Wilbur Cohen in the mid 1960s, when John W. Gardner was Secretary of the Department. The professional health responsibilities of the Surgeon General were transferred in what was called Reorganization Plan Number 3, to the Secretary of Health, Education, and Welfare. The "coup de grace" was given in April 1968, when direct authority for the Public Health Service was assigned to the Assistant Secretary for Health and Scientific Affairs and the Surgeon General[1] was designated as his deputy. The latter was also stripped of his staff responsibility for such tasks as program analysis, budget, and personnel administration. That decision had two immediate detrimental effects. First, it wiped out the line of professional promotion because there was no longer a top career position. Second, it subjugated the scientific and professional activities of the major public health and medical care agency of the United States to direct political domination.

The results were predictable. Members of the top echelon of professional personnel in the Public Health Service resigned or retired and took up new positions in universities, in industry, and in other governmental agencies. To fill the power vacuum, the major top-level vacant positions were filled one by one not on the basis of

1. This evaluation is concerned with improving the effectiveness of the scientific and professional components of public health and medical care administration in the United States and is not a defense of the quasi-military status of the United States Public Health Service.

professional competence and experience but primarily because of the political affiliation of the appointee and his acceptability to those responsible for the domestic program in the Office of the President. Even the position of the Director of the National Institutes of Health, the top medical scientific post in our government, became, with the enactment of the Cancer Control Act of 1971, a straight political appointment without any specified scientific or professional qualification. Moreover, the turnover of major professional and scientific personnel within those posts has been so rapid that institutional memory has been lost. New appointees have great difficulty in determing their exact role in maintaining the health of the country. As a result, political expediency, not professional and scientific knowledge and judgment, has become the basis for major decisions affecting the health of the country.

The harm resulting from the elimination of scientific and professional competence as the main criterion for appointment to the top administrative posts in health and medical care has been aggravated by the change in the method of allocation of federal health funds to states and local communities. Federal grants to states for example, for the care of crippled children were made by the Children's Bureau subject to built-in standards. Now those grants are being replaced by revenue-sharing, the block allocation of funds, without any scientific or professional guidelines. It has taken more than half a century of national voluntary and governmental efforts to establish standards and guidelines which through federal grants have gradually built up the effectiveness of local health services throughout the United States. Indeed, the guidelines are the distillate of the knowledge and wisdom of the most prestigious scientists and physicians in medicine and public health. It is very unlikely that such competence will be available to guide every state and metropolis in the United States as each goes its own way in developing its own local public health programs.

If major medical decisions such as the unbalanced allocation of funds for health purposes in the President's health budget and the frenetic attempts of the Congress to restore the cuts in the budget for 1973–1974 continue to be made on the basis of political expedience and not of actual need, I fear that much unnecessary disease, disability, and untimely death will have to occur throughout the country before the public becomes aware and demands that health and medical care decisions be based on the practical and efficient implementation of scientific knowledge, professional competence, technical skills, and institutional resources. It is indeed unfortunate that at this critical stage in the evolution of a national health and medical care program, our national government is so ill prepared to meet the challenge.

The Recommended Model

The Congress will soon enact legislation to create a national health and medical care program. Whatever form the new program takes, the national agency responsible for administration must be able to solve the inherent scientific, professional, organizational, and political problems. The first essential step in the inauguration of such a program must be the rebirth and development of an effective national health and medical care administration.

The recommended model is that of health administration in the United Kingdom. Provision is made in that model for a separation of the political from the professional and scientific aspects of health administration and for their balanced interaction. In the Ministry of Health and Social Security in the United Kingdom, the Minister and his immediate aides are politicians, appointed by the government in power, who are properly concerned with the political aspects of the health services. Within the ministry, a Chief Medical Officer of Health heads up a cadre of qualified career personnel, who, together with a battery of part-time advisors from universities and research institutes, are responsible for the scientific and professional aspects of public health and medical care. The Chief Medical Officer for Health works in tandem with a professional administrator who has the title of Permanent Secretary. The relative continuity and solidity of this professional unit are attested to by the fact that since the beginning of World War II the United Kingdom has had sixteen different Ministers of Health but only three Chief Medical Officers of Health.

This record is in sharp contrast with the American experience. For example, the United States lacked a chief health administrator for the entire first half of 1969, as a result of the political controversy that prevented the appointment of Dr. John H. Knowles as Assistant Secretary for Health.

The Implementation

The structure of the Department of Health, Education, and Welfare permits the development of an administrative mechanism in the United States similar to that of the United Kingdom. The political component of health administration would be concentrated in the Office of the Secretary, and the scientific, professional, and technical components would be integrated in a unit which I shall call the National Health Service. I hold no brief for any particular title for the unit or its director. But in the light of the recent history of constantly changing administrative structure and responsibilities and authority for health services at the national level, the reestablishment of the titles of the United States Public Health Service and Surgeon General for the professional, scientific, and technical unit and its director might be confusing and could handicap the evolution of the new program and the recruitment of high calibre scientific and professional personnel. It is probably better to start afresh. For the purposes of this blueprint, I shall use the title of Chief Medical Officer for the director of the National Health Service.

Liaison arrangements must be precise enough to favor the close coordination and interaction of these two essential aspects (political and professional) of public health and medical care administration. The Secretary and his aides, including the Assistant Secretary for Health, would be responsible for the political aspects of health administration. They would work closely with the Office of the President and other departments and units in the Executive Branch, with Congress and its commit-

The Implementation 249

Figure 4. Administrative structure for a national health program.

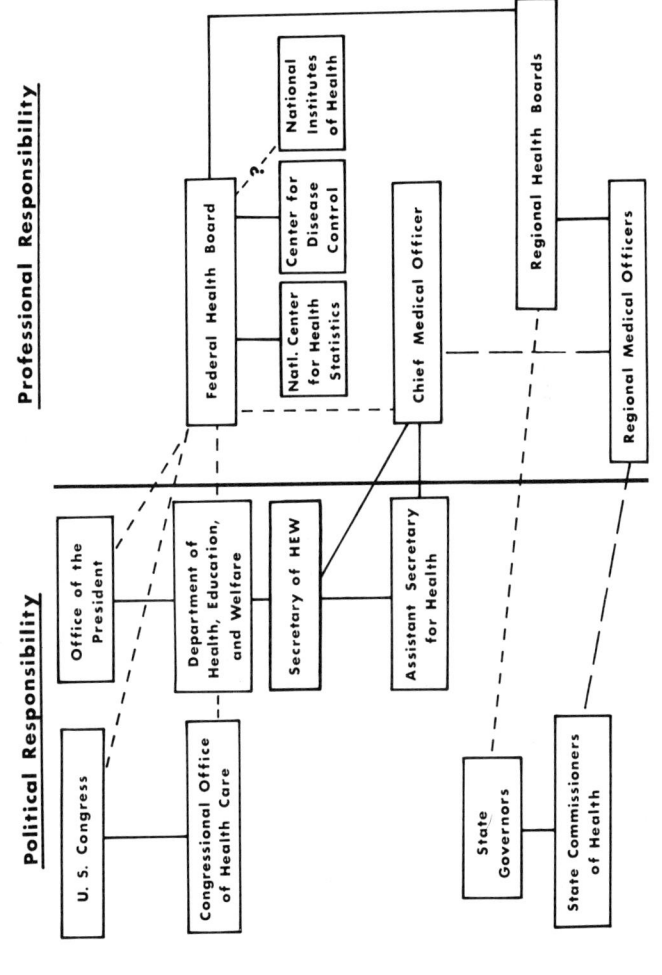

tees, and with the public at large. Health education of the public would be facilitated by the Congressional Office of Health, which would be responsible for the surveillance of the particular aspects of health and medical care that should be of immediate public interest. It would also serve as a channel of communication between the government and the public at large.

Within the Department of Health, Education, and Welfare, the National Health Service would be headed by the Chief Medical Officer, an outstanding medical administrator responsible to the Secretary. Upon recommendation of the Secretary, he would be appointed by the President with the approval of the Senate. To overlap presidential tenure, the term of office would be at least six years and reappointment would be unlimited until the mandatory retirement age. The National Health Service would comprise all existing bureaus of the Department of Health, Education, and Welfare that have direct medical care responsibilities. Other health administrative entities, including the Food and Drug Administration and the National Library of Medicine, would probably be kept separate but this would be a matter for administrative decision. It is moot whether the intensive medical research arm of the government, the National Institutes of Health, should remain within the Department of Health, Education, and Welfare or should become affiliated with the Federal Health Board. The latter arrangement would provide for close liaison with the quality control system, including the National Center for Health Statistics and the Center for Disease Control, within the Federal Health Board. In any event, the National Health Service in the Department of Health, Education, and Welfare would have to work very closely with the Federal Health Board on the scientific, professional, and technical aspects of providing to the people high quality medical care as efficiently as possible.

Local Health Administration

The unit of local health administration is the medical care region as previously defined. All local health units now existing within each region would be combined into a single regional health authority. There are many precedents for such integration in classic state health department programs as, for example, in the grouping of counties in New York State and of towns in Massachusetts into health districts. State legislation may be needed to provide the legal basis for the regional health units. Prior to the inauguration of a national health program, the governor of each state, working with the state health department, would recommend to the state legislature the necessary changes in state public health law (and, when appropriate, in the state sanitary code by the public health council or board of health), so that local health administrative units can be brought together into medical care regions.

In each medical care region, a regional health board would be established, the members of which would be appointed upon the advice of the state commissioner of health by the governor within standards established by the Federal Health Board and with its approval. Each medical care region would be administered by a regional medical officer. Since the medical care program will be federally financed, the regional medical officer would be nominated by the regional health board and appointed by the Chief Medical Officer in the Department of Health, Education, and Welfare. The line of administration would run from the Secretary through the Chief Medical Officer in the Department of Health, Education, and Welfare to the regional medical officer in the medical care region. But when the police and regulatory powers of the state are involved, as in the control of epidemics or in assuring the safety of the environment, the regional medical officer would be responsible to the state health commissioner.

The recommended administrative structure is straightforward enough when the medical care region is located entirely within the state. Where medical service areas with their established marketing patterns and communication and transportation systems overlap state boundary lines—southern New Jersey, for example, centers on Philadelphia—the medical care regional administration would have to be set up jointly by the authorities of both states. Where major problems override state boundary lines, there are many precedents for the establishment of such interstate authorities, as in the New England River Basins Commission.

In metropolitan areas, where many medical schools and teaching hospitals are located and where many health regions would come together, it would be a matter of local decision as to whether the health regions would be administered separately or in groups.

In summary, the regional medical officer and the regional medical board, the policy-making group, working together and affiliated at the national level with the Department of Health, Education, and Welfare, the Federal Health Board, and the Congressional Office of Health Care, would be responsible for the administration of each regional medical care program.

Financing Medical Care 18

The Insurance Principle
In the United States, except for a relatively few complete medical care programs, the financing of most medical care on the insurance principle has been perforce limited in scope. Most plans, whether they are insured by Blue Cross-Blue Shield, private insurance companies, or governmental agencies, have had to focus on reimbursement for inpatient services because physician services in ambulatory care are for the most part uninsurable. This tendency has increased the total cost of care. Patients who would be better treated as ambulatory cases are, for purposes of insurance coverage, admitted to the expensive inpatient services of hospitals for diagnostic procedures. As a result, we establish and support many more hospital beds in the United States than we really need.

Why can't we insure for ambulatory care in the United States? The answer is very simple. Insurance risks must be predictable. We have already seen that the open-ended system of fee-for-service payment makes it impossible to calculate either the total cost of physician services or an annual insurance premium. The cost of one segment of physician's care, that of inpatient services, is more predictable because of built-in controls. These include the fixed number of hospital beds, the screening process in hospital admission, the hospital utilization committees that supervise the use of hospital beds, and the regulations of the Commission on Hospital Accreditation that limit the performance of unnecessary procedures within the hospital. It is obvious that none of these controls is applicable to physician services in our catch-as-catch-can nonsystem of ambulatory medical care. If a national health program is to insure for complete medical care in a defined budget, the physician must be paid by a method, such as the one proposed in this blueprint, in which total annual cost is predictable.

Federal Insurance
Recent experience with the Kerr-Mills and Medicaid programs as contrasted with Medicare makes it crystal clear that the financing of a national medical care program must be solely a federal and not a joint federal-state effort. The Kerr-Mills program and its offspring, Medicaid, were established by Congressional legislation, but they both require separate implementing legislation and annual appropriations out of general funds in each of the fifty states. As state legislatures have dragged their feet, those programs have constantly been bound down by red tape and have operated unequally throughout the country. The wide variation in coverage

has on the average favored the residents of the richer states with more extensive benefits, while some states have provided no benefits at all. In contrast, the Medicare program, financed directly through the federal Social Security Administration, has insured uniform benefits in somewhat more efficient fashion to all eligible aged citizens throughout the country.

Medicare and Medicaid are both incomplete programs and their deductions and exclusions and limitations of benefits are almost incomprehensible. The patient does not understand that payment for services are based not on his needs but on the insurability of individual procedures. He becomes even more confused when he learns that the benefits of Medicare and Medicaid are not the same. In attempting to discover why certain costs of his recent illness were not covered, he is forced to deal with a faceless bureaucracy that knows nothing about his illness and little about the reasons for the exclusions. The frustrations and the financial complexities of the incomplete Medicare and Medicaid programs have created an urgent need for an ombudsman, as expensive as that might be, to serve as a friend in court for the patient. Until a national health program is established, the services of an ombudsman are essential to unwind the red tape and to find the best solution to each patient's problem. In their turn, the physician, the hospital, and other purveyors of service have also been dissatisfied because of the unnecessary complexity of administration and the long delays in the payment for care.

The spiraling costs of medical care whether financed nationally (Medicare) or jointly (Medicaid) have forced progressive cuts in health benefits to the insured in order to keep the total costs of the programs within finite limits. If a comprehensive national health program is not established, this immutable trend must eventually reach the point where enormous expenditures of funds will provide very little medical care. The national administration and the Congress, as well as the state governments, have studiously avoided facing up to the two underlying reasons for this trend toward bankruptcy—the failure of hospitals to define and live within fixed annual budgets, and the open-ended, uninsurable fee-for-service system of physician payment. Our political representatives will have to come to grips with this issue if all Americans are to have the benefits of modern medicine.

The complete medical care plan proposed in this blueprint will do away with many of these vexing problems because of the relative simplicity of its financing and payment mechanisms. Exclusions and limitations of benefits to those served by the program will be reduced to a minimum, and purveyors will not have to be reimbursed individually for each procedure and service. The new system would relieve the recipients of care of the constant haggling over approval of payments, and the purveyors of care would be spared mountains of paperwork and the financial losses associated with delayed reimbursement. As a result, the hypertrophic bureaucracy now responsible for Medicare and Medicaid administration would be trimmed down to size and the funds thereby recovered could be applied to the prevention and treatment of disease.

Proposed Method of Financing
This blueprint of a single uniform national medical care program requires a method of financing that meets the following criteria: (1) the total annual cost of the program will be determined by the Congress from budget requests of the Department of Health, Education, and Welfare as approved by the Office of Management and Budget and as based upon the professional and technical advice and the priority lists established by the Federal Health Board, and will aim to satisfy the public interest as expressed through the Congressional Office of Health; (2) all medical care costs are to be prepaid on the insurance principle; (3) a single uniform system of insurance will simplify administration and accounting and will eliminate the unnecessary expense of keeping track of the almost limitless number of heterogeneous, variable, and incomplete insurance programs; (4) the insurance system must operate directly and uniformly between the federal government and the individual or the family without the delays, obstructions, and unequal treatment created by the implementing state legislation, as in Medicaid, or the awkwardness and additional expense of middleman administration, as by Blue Cross-Blue Shield in the Medicare program; (5) annual contributions of the individual or family should be made in accordance with ability to pay, with supplements from general funds to cover the unemployed and the unemployable; (6) coinsurance payments—small direct payment by the patient at the time he receives the service—are essential to foster a sense of participation by the beneficiaries and to eliminate nuisance calls, but they

must be severely restricted whenever they might create a barrier to medical care and are therefore to be avoided entirely for preventive services, for the treatment of the early stages of potentially serious disease, and for chronic disabling or catastrophic illness.

Except for adjustment of individual contributions to ability to pay, the Social Security tax could be the best method of financing. But the Social Security tax is as retrogressive as a sales tax and bears most heavily upon those with smaller incomes. Moreover, in recent years it has been constantly increased to meet the cost of new benefits and to keep up with inflation. The Social Security tax is now so close to its maximum tolerable level that it is highly unlikely that the cost of the proposed national health program could be met from that source. Nevertheless, a small proportion of the cost should be covered by the Social Security tax because it is desirable that each person realize that he is making a direct payment for his medical care.

During the past few decades, industrial labor contracts have been a major source of health insurance funds. It is a retrogressive tax, but it would be wise to continue to tap that source for a limited fraction of the cost of the total program. A one-percent tax on industrial payrolls, paid for by industry as in the past, would seem reasonable.

Finally, we turn to the federal income tax. The federal income tax with its progressive rates most closely relates the amount of the tax to ability to pay. Moreover, it is the most effective federal tax and most of the cost of medical care for the entire population will have to be met from that source.

The Social Security Administration would be responsible for managing the insurance and the fiscal aspects of the national health program. It would be responsible for assembling the funds to meet the total cost of the program, from the Social Security tax, the payroll tax, the supplements from general funds for the medically indigent, the coinsurance payments, and the income tax. The Social Security Administration would also handle all disbursements through its nationwide administrative structure. It must be understood that assignment of these responsibilities to the Social Security Administration would not authorize that agency to administer the total program. The national health program would be administered by the Office of the Assistant Secretary and the Chief Medical Officer of the Department of Health, Education, and Welfare in collaboration with the Federal Health Board and the Congressional Office of Health Care.

Public acceptance of financing the national health program by tax payments is crucial to its success. Acceptance will be fostered by the knowledge that the tax payments for the new program will replace and will not be in addition to the more than eighty billion dollars expended annually in the country for medical care. Each person must be made aware of how much he now pays out of pocket for his medical care in the form of health insurance premiums, payments to physicians and hospitals, taxes to support Medicare, Medicaid, municipal and state hospitals and institutions, and other governmental programs, expenditures for prosthetic devices and other health services, not to mention the bankrupting drain of catastrophic illness. He must understand that the introduction of the national health program would relieve him of all of these payments. The taxpayer will be further persuaded to pay for medical care through the tax mechanism by a clear demonstration of the savings that will accrue to him and to his family from the prevention of unnecessary disease, the warding off of unnecessary disability, and the postponement of untimely death that can be achieved by replacement of existing medical care by a quality controlled national health program. The Department of Health, Education, and Welfare—the administrator of the national health program—and its regional affiliates must perform the economic and fiscal analyses to provide information to the public about the sparing effect of a national health program on personal expenditures for medical care, and to weld that information into an effective educational program for the people of the country.

The Crucial Question

19

This blueprint for medical care, even in its preliminary form, promises many benefits that could improve our national health. Constructive criticisms and suggestions will favor the evolution of the proposed plan, whose final form must depend on rigorous testing through mathematical models, simulation on the computer, and controlled experiments in the field. An enormous amount of work must be done, but the potential rewards justify the effort.

A sound and feasible plan does not by itself guarantee better health for anyone. Success will depend ultimately on the answer to the following question: How can our complex society suppress its primitive fears of change and use our treasure of existing knowledge, our army of educated and trained personnel, our superb institutional structures, our rapidly expanding technology, and our storehouse of social and financial resources, and rally the providers and consumers of medical care on the basis of enlightened self-interest to diminish suffering, postpone untimely death, and improve our individual and national health?

The answer is specific, but accomplishment will be difficult. We need brilliant, strong, and vigorous leadership buttressed with the statesmanship to decide what must be done. We need the political acumen to convert hope into reality. We need an educational program for the providers and the consumers of medical care to give them the information they must have for the selection of able representatives who can do the job. The opportunities to improve the health of the people are all around us. Will we take advantage of them?

Appendix

Physicians for Americans
Two Medical Curricula: a New Proposal*

David D. Rutstein

A prime responsibility of medical schools is to educate enough of the different kinds of physicians needed to provide adequate medical care for the people. . . .

The number of physicians now practising in the United States, and those to be graduated during the next decade, do not and cannot meet the needs of our growing and changing population if demands for medical service continue at the present level. . . .

The growing deficiency is greater among those providing general medical services—i.e., general practitioners, internists, and pediatricians. . . . This trend towards the disappearance of the general physician is nation-wide. It is shown by the complete lack of physician's services in some rural areas and the shift toward specialty practice in urban areas. . . .

When a patient has no general physician, lack of continuity in his medical care is inevitable. His health

* Abstracted from *The Lancet*, March 4, 1961, pp. 498–501.

will not be properly supervised and gaps will occur in his care when he is ill. Moreover, he is often confused by conflicting information given to him as he goes from specialist to specialist or is referred from one service to another in our highly compartmentalised hospitals. . . .

Not into General Practice

It is clear why graduates of American medical schools tend not to go into general practice. Since the Flexner report, the medical schools have pursued a policy which favours the education of experts—i.e., scientists and specialists—rather than general physicians. This policy was aided and abetted by:

1. The high priority given by medical-school admission committees to applicants with demonstrated scientific ability.
2. A medical-school curriculum concentrating on minutiæ of preclinical science sometimes at the expense of clinical teaching.
3. The preferential appointment by our great teaching hospitals of interns and residents with scientific ability rather than those with clinical acumen.
4. The appointment of scientists interested in research in one of the preclinical sciences instead of clinicians as heads of clinical departments.
5. The availability of large sums for medical research with a concomitant lack of financial support for medical education.
6. The development of the specialty boards.

Appendix

And last but not least,

7. The patient's immediate acceptance of and willingness to pay for the services of the specialist.

The policy of producing highly qualified scientists and specialists must continue. It has been responsible for the flowering and the excellent reputation of American medicine. We must be sure that the highly specialised research programme of our medical schools be stimulated and expanded if we are to remain in the vanguard of those contributing to medical advance. Students now being educated in ever-narrowing fields will not only contribute to research—they will also use their highly specialised knowledge and techniques for the patient's benefit.

But, at the same time, this policy has created new and serious gaps in general medical care. The educational needs of the specialist and scientist on the one hand and general physicians on the other grow farther and farther apart, and it is increasingly difficult to include them within the compass of the medical curriculum. The low-ranking student who cannot make the grade in our research-oriented curriculum drifts off into general practice. This raises a most serious question. How can the medical schools continue to provide top medical scientists and at the same time graduate competent physicians in numbers adequate to meet our medical care needs?

When we examine the situation closely, we realise that the compromise reached by our present medical curriculum does an injustice both to the education of the expert as well as to that of the general physician. As has been pointed out in the studies by Helen Gee,* the medical student body is a heterogeneous group both in ability and motivation. In our attempts to reach this broad spectrum of students, we have been forced on the one hand to teach the expert at too elementary a level while presenting an overspecialised curriculum to the future general physician. . . . These compromises will continue to impair the future of medical science and of medical care in the United States as long as we depend upon a single medical curriculum to do both jobs.

A Way Out

A possible way out of this impasse is to follow the lead of schools of technology such as the Massachusetts Institute of Technology. They have recognised that the educational needs of the physicist and the engineer are different. Although students entering these fields may start off together, their curricula diverge. This is not to say that a student selecting one of these may not change to the other if he so decides and if his qualifications permit. Students with a special interest may also select elective courses in the other curriculum.

In medicine a similar programme is possible. Two curricula can be designed—one for research-workers, specialists, and future professors and the other for general physicians. For purposes of discussion and debate, I will

* H. H. Gee, "Differential Characteristics of Student Bodies in Selection and Educational Differentiation," report of a conference held May 25–27, 1959, at the University of California: p. 125.

Appendix

give examples of the curricular changes which illustrate the principles which might be followed if a two-curricula system were adopted.

The research specialist curriculum must include more instruction in the newer preclinical sciences and in mathematics. For example, recent developments in physics, electrical engineering, and mathematics open new pathways to important medical knowledge not accessible to conventional research methods. At the present time, most clinical research tends to be limited to the study of first-order reactions—i.e., one-to-one relationships. Now, application of mathematical theory makes it possible to interpret complex interrelated systems such as that of the absorption of fats from the intestine where splitting and recombination of compounds and recirculation take place simultaneously. Or, through multivariant analysis it is now possible to study the function of a complex organ such as the kidney. Also, newer mathematical models of physiological functions such as that of muscular contraction now provide better hypotheses for the inductive scientist to test in his experiments. In biochemical research, mathematical analysis of randomly split peptide fragments now makes possible the determination of the order of aminoacids in a protein, thus shortcutting the painfully slow process of splitting linkages with specific enzymes.

Such newer knowledge will also assist the specialist in his care of patients. For example, analysis of electronic records as has been demonstrated by Pipberger for the electrocardiogram gives promise of relieving cardiologists of the routine reading and the interpretation of tracings. These newer developments in medical research and in specialty practice have been abetted by the continuing development of computation systems and the increasing availability of such equipment.

Therefore, the curriculum for the student looking toward a career in medical research or in specialty practice must include enough mathematics, physics, and electrical engineering to enable him to work effectively in research teams on which PH.D. scientists in these fields will be represented. This is similar to the present need of the clinical investigator for a basic knowledge of biochemistry. Depending upon individual interests, students will have to learn enough mathematics to handle problems concerned with probability theory, must master differential and integral calculus, and in many cases differential equations—enough electrical engineering to use this growing technology in the design of the experiments and enough understanding of physics to incorporate current theory in the study of such phenomena as perception. Time for such study can be made available by shortening of the clinical teaching in specialties not in the field of the student's interest, permitting many more elective courses, and if necessary, lengthening of the curriculum in particular fields. Thus, a student looking forward to a future in research on perception may spend more time in ophthalmology and less in genitourinary diseases, while one interested in the research on the physiology of the kidney might reverse his selections. Certainly, education of the general physician in a

Appendix

different curriculum will add flexibility to the curriculum of the clinical research-worker and the specialist.

The curriculum for the general physician should be shorter than the present one. Condensed medical curricula compressing college and medical school instruction in a six-year course have been proposed by Johns Hopkins University, Northwestern University, and Boston University. It is difficult to see how such a single condensed curriculum can be satisfactory both for the scientist and the general physician when the present longer one is not. But, such a condensed curriculum would lend itself to the education of the general physician at about the level of our present internist. With such a shortened curriculum many more doctors could be educated than under the present system. This assumes, of course, that there also would be a curriculum for the education of the scientist and the specialist.

More Selective Education

The key to the new curriculum for the general physician is selectivity of those scientific facts and theories germane to his particular task. That task consists of the general supervision of health and medical care, including preventive medicine, the treatment of minor illnesses, the practice of minor surgery and perhaps normal obstetrics, and the screening of patients for early manifestations of severe or chronic illness in which early treatment gives a better prognosis or a more comfortable life.

Much time in the present curriculum is devoted to learning an almost infinite number of details, many of which are not needed by the general physician. For example, during my medical-school education, I was expected to learn the origin and insertion of all of the striated muscles of the body. This was the era of the anatomist—gross, microscopic, or morbid. When his influence declined, with the rise of biochemistry, this anatomical requirement was deleted from the medical curriculum. But, instead, students are expected to learn, in the same unselective way, the names and functions of all the enzymes in all the known chemical reactions in the muscles of the body. To be sure, knowledge of the principles of enzyme action and of the Krebs cycle is important and should be taught to the general physician. But, the details of the individual chemical reactions, of great interest to the biochemist and the expert in metabolism, do not concern him.

Just as research has become more complex, so has medical care. The evolution of the specialist in medicine, the increasing use of clinical and other laboratories, and the many paramedical assistants all demand a general physician who knows how to interrelate all of these essential services for the benefit of a particular patient. Moreover, the increasing burden of chronic disease associated with lengthening life-expectancy demands more detailed supervision of the individual patient. This is so whether the patient is cared for by the specialist services of the hospital or at home with the assistance of community health services. The curriculum of the general physician, therefore, must include time for the detailed supervision of, for example, the ambulatory cancer patient whose treatment may require at particular times a surgeon, a radiologist, or radiotherapist, a specialist in metabolism, an anæsthesiologist to control his pain, the psychiatrist, selected laboratory tests, or the services of a public-health nurse, medical social worker, dietitian, or physiotherapist.

Most important of all, the general physician must have had special teaching on the theory and technique of screening patients for early manifestations of those serious or chronic illnesses which are better treated early. Under his general supervision, he must be able to refer patients, so identified, to proper treatment even though it require a particular specialist, an unusual laboratory test, or a service to be given by a member of one of the paramedical professions. This means that the clinical competence of the general physician must be excellent. The curriculum must stress clinical instruction particularly on patients in the early stages of illness.

These are representative examples of the kind of curricular changes that would be possible if the two-curricula system were adopted. Depending upon his special field of medical education the teacher can visualise the changes which would improve his teaching programme if the additional flexibility of a two-curricula system were made available.

If a two-curricula system were adopted, there would be another advantage. The medical schools could have a more selective admission policy. Candidates for admission to the research-specialist curriculum would be expected to have different qualifications from those applying for the general-physician curriculum. The former should attract the kind of student who has been turning away from medicine towards a career in mathematics or in such sciences as physics and chemistry.

In contrast, the general physician's curriculum should attract some of those dedicated and able students who have hesitated to apply or have been frightened away from medical school because of their inability to compete at an advanced level with those more gifted in the sciences. It would be a great novelty to see the top man in a medical-school class yearning to be the best physician rather than the best scientist.

Costs of Gains
Increased recruitment will have to be supported by extension to medicine of such scholarship aid programmes as the pre-doctoral fellowship programmes of the federal government. Large sums for building and the operation of medical schools will also be needed. It should be pointed out, however, that there is no reason why this particular plan should cost more than other plans for expansion of medical schools. Indeed, by shortening the education curriculum for general physicians, it should cost less.

Recruitment of faculty for this proposed programme should be less difficult than recruitment for a mere expansion of the present medical schools. As in the latter case, more scientists will have to be recruited for preclinical teaching. However, for clinical teaching an unused resource could be tapped. Many skilful young clinicians in our teaching hospitals now have no academic future because they are not adept at laboratory research. Many are now forced unwillingly into private practice. They would make excellent full-time clinical professors, many of whom will be needed if we develop a curriculum directed toward the education of the general physician.

Two Curricula but One School
One point must be clear. My suggestion for reorganising medical education provides for two curricula in the same medical school and not for different curricula in separate schools. This latter system, which I oppose, would have two major defects. It would educate medical scientists in an environment where there would be insufficient exposure to the problems of clinical medicine demanding thoroughgoing research. But, more important, it would result in vocational schools for general physicians. As in the case of the present education of the internist, the curriculum for the general physician must be soundly based on medical science in a school where the student is in close contact not only with clinical teachers but also with research-workers and specialists. To do otherwise would bring a rapid return of all of the evils of the pre-Flexner era. . . .

Index

Academic freedom in health care systems, 212
Administrative record system, 33–34
Administrative structure of a national health program, 242–252
organization chart, 249
Allied health personnel, 22–24, 57–61, 105, 109–112, 128, 231
in reception center, 95, 120
in treatment center, 99, 101
professional education of, 35–36
Ambulances, 71–74
Ambulatory care, 80–102
clinics, 86–87, 93–97
at community hospital, 99–102
for disadvantaged populations, 87–90
essential elements of, 98–99
group practice, 84–85
institutional, 86–87
patient referral system in, 120–123
private, 82–85
treatment centers, 93–97
American Cancer Society, 165
American College of Physicians, 164
American College of Surgeons, 164
American Foundation for Negro Affairs, 157
American Heart Association, 165
American Medical Association, 52, 243
American Nurses Association, 52, 56
American Society of Medical Technologists, 52
Ayres, W. R., 31n

Bartley, M. A., 157n
Bedford V.A. Hospital, 38, 40
Bell Laboratories, 45
Blacklow, R. S., 156n
Boston University Medical Center, 47
Brown University Medical School, 47
Burke, F. G., 31n

Cancer program, 200, 202, 214
Captain of the team, *see* General physician
Carnegie Commission on Higher Education, 39, 50, 57, 147n

Index

Castelli, W. P., 73n
Center for Disease Control, 12, 26, 48, 172, 179–180, 186, 188–190, 192, 193, 199, 200, 201, 206, 213, 250
  current program summarized, 193
Charts
  figure 1, The hospital of the future, 6
  figure 2, A regional system, 16
  figure 3, Ambulatory care, 49
  figure 4, Administrative structure for a national health program, 249
Chief medical officer of the United States, 248–250
Children's Bureau, 243, 245
Clinical research, 31–32
  studies to measure outcome, 166
Clinics, ambulatory care, 86–87
  freestanding, 93–96
  hospital-connected, 96–97
Closed-circuit television, 38–41, 44
Code, national health, 220–222
Cohen, Wilbur, 244
College of General Practitioners, 164
Columbia Point Program, Boston, 88
Commission on Hospital Accreditation, 165, 255
Communication and transportation, 133–138
  engineering and technology, 133–135
  planning, 136
Communications system, 36–37, 133–138
  in ambulatory care, 121–122
  electronic communication in medical care, 37–45
  electronic signals, 36
  in emergency care, 69–71
  engineering, 135–137
  in reception center, 121
  in regional system, 20, 44–46
Computer, use of
  in diagnosis, 125–127
  tickler files, 129
Computer simulation studies
  in distribution of hospital activities, 19, 21
Confidential record system, 30, 32, 167
Congressional Office of Health Care, 210–212, 213, 219, 258
  liaison with Federal Health Board, 210–211, 222–223
  responsible for surveillance, 250
  watchdog function of, 226–228
Congressional Office of Technology Assessment, 227
Consultation at a distance, 37–46
  instruments needed for, 41–43
  Picturephone, 45
  television, 38–41, 44–45
Continuity of care, 24, 102, 106
Converting to a national health program, 209–213
  order of procedure, 211–212
Cost of medical care, 137–138, 228, 260
  exponential rise in, 203, 256
  proportion of Gross National Product, 228
Crisis
  energy, 75
  environmental, 75
  rush-hour emergencies, 75–76
  transportation, 75
Crucial question, 261

Department of Health, Education, and Welfare, 65, 201, 211, 212, 213, 218, 219, 242, 248, 258, 261
  liaison with President and Congress, 248

Index

reorganization of health services, 1952, 243–245
Depersonalization of medical care, 2–3, 107–108
Diagnosis
　physician's role in, 123–125
　use of the computer in, 125–127
Disadvantaged populations, 87–90
Disadvantaged students in medical school, 155–157

Early treatment, 11, 104, 127, 177
Early warning system, 191–198, 215
Eden, Murray, 34n, 145n
Electronic communication, 36–45
Emergency aide, 67, 72
Emergency care, 62–79
　command center, 69–71
　communications system, 69–71
　essential elements of, 67
　military experience in, 66–67
　regional program for, 67–79
　transportation system, 71–76
　treatment centers, 64, 76–78
Emergency communications network, 69–71
Emergency telephones, 69
Emergency treatment center, 76–78
Emergency vehicles, 71–76
Extended care facilities, 9
Extensive vs. intensive research, 179–185

Federal grants to states, 245
Federal Health Board, 48, 199, 200–224, 258
　duties, 208–223
　liaison with Congressional Office of Health Care, 210–211, 222–223
　liaison with Department of Health, Education, and Welfare, 205, 213
　liaison with regional health boards, 207–208
　membership, 205
　not an administrative agency, 204
　structure, 205
　watchdog function, 213
Federal income tax to finance national health program, 259
Federal insurance for medical care, 255–257
Federal Reserve Board, 205
Fee-for-service payment, 237–238
Filer, D. C., 13n
Financing medical care, 254–261
　generating public acceptance, 260–261
　through federal insurance, 255, 258–259
　through federal taxes, 259
　through payroll tax, 259
First aid, 130–131
Flexner medical curriculum, 139, 140
Food and Drug Administration, 201, 243, 250
Framingham Heart Study, 73–74

Gardner, John W., 244
General physician, 103–118
　as captain of the team, 3, 53, 104–118
　decline, 112, 265–267
　hospital-based, 115–116
　medical education of, 157–158, 268–274
　medical school curriculum for, 159–160, 265–275
　rebirth, 114–116
　relationship with specialist, 105–107, 112–114, 116–118

Index

General physician (*continued*)
  responsibility for total care, 104–110, 116–118
  scarcity, 83, 90
  services provided by, 104–109
Gordon, Myron, 32n
Group Health Association, 85
Group practice, 8, 84–85
  defined, 85
Guidance system, 175–191, 215
  feasibility, 189
  implementation, 185–189
  prerequisites, 190–191

Harvard Careers Summer Program, 156
Harvard Medical School, 36
  core curriculum, 141–142
  Flexner curriculum, 139, 140
  hospital complex, 47
Health administration
  local, 251–253
  national, 242–251
  organization chart, 249
Health alerting system, 232–235
Health, Education, and Welfare, Department of, *see* Department of Health, Education, and Welfare
Health officer, local
  duties, 234
  merged with hospital administrator, 10
Health Research Institute of the City of New York, 213
Heartmobile, 65, 73
Helicopter, 65, 74–75
Home visiting services, 131–132
Hospital, central, 17, 20–26, 48–49
  elements of care, 17
Hospital, community, 5–14, 48–49
  elements of care, 11
  in regional system, 15–26
Hospital, cottage, 17–19

integration with community hospital, 19
  in Sweden, 18
Hospital, regional, 15–26
Hospital, teaching, 15–17, 35, 47
Hospital administrator
  duties, 234
  merged with local health officer, 10
Hospital of the future, 7–14
  chart, 6
Hospital standards, 165–166
Hospital training, 145

Incentive awards to the physician, 239–241
Income tax, federal, 259
Indices of health
  existing, 169–173
  infant mortality, 170–172
  life expectancy, 170–172
  new, 214–216
Information clearing house, 34
Information processing, 27–34
Institute of Medicine, 206
Institutional care
  ambulatory, 8, 86–87
  emergency, 77–78
  inpatient, 7–8, 21–22, 105–106
  regional, 46–51
Institutional structure, 5–14
  chart, 6
Intensive care, 21–22
Intensive vs. extensive research, 179–185

Kaiser-Permanente Program, 167, 240
Kennedy, Senator Robert F., 64
Kerr-Mills program, 255
Knowles, Dr. John, 247

Laboratory specimens, transporting, 24–26

Index

Landrigan, P. J., 197n
Licensure of physicians
  examinations, 163
  laws, 52–54
Local health administration, 251–253
Luchsinger, P. 31n

McNamara, Patricia, 73n
Marketing areas and regional health care, 17, 207–208, 251
  see also Medical service areas
Martin Luther King Program, Bronx, New York, 88
Massachusetts Eye and Ear Infirmary, 68
Massachusetts General Hospital, 38, 40, 47
  Family Health Program, 70
Massachusetts Medical Society, 171
Medicaid, 164, 255–256, 257, 258
Medical care
  essential components of, 103–104
  quality distinct from efficiency, 161–163, 168–169
Medical care region, 251
  defined, 46–47
  and local marketing area, 17, 207–208, 251
Medical corpsman, see Military medical corpsman
Medical education, 139–160
  continuity, 147–149
  core curriculum, 140–142
  criteria for medical curriculum, 143–144
  disadvantaged students, 155–157
  flexibility, 146, 151–152
  Flexner curriculum, 139, 140
  multichannel curriculum, 141–152
  qualifications for admission, 152–158

Medical manpower, 52–60
Medical military corpsman, see Military medical corpsman
Medical records
  computerized record system, 29–31
  confidentiality, 30, 32, 167
  confusion in, 28–29
  disposable, 30
  record-linkage system, 29
Medical Research Council of Great Britain, 179, 180
Medical school teaching hospital, see Hospital, teaching
Medical service areas, 46–51
  reception center in the heart of, 119
  see also Marketing areas and regional health care
Medical social worker, 108
Medical triage, see Triage
Medicare, 256, 257, 258
Mental illness, 9–10
Military experience in emergency care, 66–67
Military medical corpsman, 56, 65, 67, 72
Muirhead, D. M., 171n
Multichannel medical curriculum
  continuity, 147–149
  criteria, 143–144
  pathways, 144–145
Murray, D. B., 31n

National Academy of Sciences, 64–65, 201, 206
National Board of Medical Examiners, 52
National Center for Health Statistics, 48, 179–180, 183, 185, 187–190, 192, 199, 200, 206, 213, 250
National health administration, 242–251

Index

National health administration (*continued*)
  organization chart, 249
National health code, 220–222
National Health Service, United Kingdom, 212–213, 247–248, 250
National Health Service, United States, 248–251
National Institutes of Health, 200–202, 213, 219, 245, 250
National Library of Medicine, 250
National Research Council, 201
National specialty boards, 53
New York Academy of Medicine, 188
Niswander, K. R., 32n
Northeastern University, 36
Nurse-midwife, 30, 55, 131
Nursing homes, 9, 12
Nyswander, D. B., 130n

Office of Management and Budget, 218, 219, 258
Office of Science and Technology, 201
Office of Vocational Rehabilitation, 243

Paramedical personnel, *see* Allied health personnel
Patient referral system, 120–123
Patient scheduling, 32–33
Payment to the physician, 236–241
  incentive awards, 239–241
  salary, 238
Peer review, 164–165
Personalized care, 3, 108–109
  see also Physician-patient relationship
Physician, general, *see* General physician

Physician, private
  unavailability, 82–83
Physician-patient relationship, 108–110, 168
  see also Personalized care
Physician's assistant, 110–112, 122, 125, 127
Physician's role, 53, 58–61
Physician's time, use of, 53–61
  see also Professional time, conserving
Picturephone, 45
Political decisions for health reasons, 201
  immunization, 201
Political pressure on health decisions, 200–201, 245–246
  cancer program, 200, 202
  Food and Drug Administration, 201
  National Institutes of Health, 201
  sickle cell anemia, 200
Politics, the art of the possible, 203
Poverty programs, 87–90
President's Manpower Commission, 57
Preventive medical care, 7, 10–11, 127–128
  at community hospital, 10
  incentive awards for, 240
  at reception center, 129
  at treatment center, 100
Priorities, recommended by Federal Health Board, 218
Privacy, protection of, 233
Professional education, 34–36, 139–160
  for allied medical professions, 35–36
  for physicians, 139–160
Professional Standards Review Organization, 165
Professional time, conserving, 22–24, 50, 57–61

Index

see also Physician's time, use of
Psychiatric care at community hospital, 9–10
Public education programs, 229–231, 235
on benefits of national health program, 260–261
on emergency care, 70
at the local level, 229–230
at the national level, 249
Public health nurse, 23–24, 105, 108
duties of, 24
in emergency care, 70
entry point to care, 234
Public Health Service of the United States, 243, 244, 248
Public interest, 225–235
at the local level, 228–229
at the national level, 226–228

Qualifications of medical personnel, 163–165
Quality control and the Federal Health Board, 213–214, 216–218, 223–224
budgetary allocation, 218–220
Quality control systems, 174–198, 223–224
early warning system, 191–198
guidance system, 175–191
Quality of medical care, 161–173
existing standards for, 163–167

Reception center, 119–132
link with medical facilities, 119
preventive services at, 119, 129
services summarized, 119–120
Regional health boards, 48, 194, 207, 212, 250
in converting to a national health program, 211
relationship with Federal Health Board, 207–208, 251

Regional medical care system, 15–26, 50–51
chart, 16
structure, 50
Regional medical officer, 251–253
Rehabilitation of the handicapped at community hospital, 11
Roles, professional, 53–61
general physician vs. specialist, 105–107, 112–114, 116–118
need for definition, 56–61
overlapping functions in, 53–55
Rutstein, D. D., 11n, 34n, 62n, 112n, 127n, 140n, 145n, 159n, 170n

Sanders, Dr. Charles, 40
School health services, 130
Screening programs, 177–179, 232
Screening tests
on ill patients, 127
in preventive care, 11
on well patients, 97, 177
Sentinel health events, 191–198
diphtheria, 197–198
identified by Center for Disease Control, 192
measles, 197–198
poliomyelitis, 197–198
Sickle cell anemia, 200
Simmons College, 36
Slow-scan television, 44
Snell, R. E., 31n
Social Security Administration, 187, 256, 260
Social Security taxes, 259
Specialist, 105, 112–114, 116-118
consultation at a distance with, 37–46
see also Superspecialist
Standards of medical care
existing, 163–167
hospital, 165–166
State governors, 251

Index

State health commissioners, 251–252
Statesmanship, the science of the necessary, 203
Stockbridge, C. D., 45n
Superspecialist, 13–14, 21, 37–46
 see also Specialist
Surgeon general, United States Public Health Service, 243, 248
Sweden, 18, 19, 33, 113, 237, 238
Systems
 ambulatory care, 92–102, 119–132; chart, 49
 communications, 20, 36–37, 69–71, 121–122, 133–138
 early warning, in quality control, 191–198
 emergency care, 62–79
 guidance, in quality control, 175–191
 health alerting, 232–235
 medical record, 29–31
 patient referral, 120–123
 quality control, 174–198
 regional, 15–26, 44–46, 50–51; chart, 16
 transportation, 133–138

Taxes to finance national health program
 federal income, 259
 industrial payroll, 259
 social security 259
Television for consultation
 closed-circuit color, 38–41, 44
 slow-scan, 44–45
Texarcana, 197
Texas, 196–198
Transportation of specimens for testing, 24–26
Transportation system, 133–138
 in ambulatory care, 122
 in emergency care, 71–76
 engineering, 135–136

 in reception center, 122
 in regional system, 20
 in Sweden, 19
Treatment center
 ambulatory, 99–102
 emergency, 64, 76–78
Triage
 in ambulatory care, 99
 defined, 66n
 in emergency care, 70, 71
 in reception center, 120
Triage nurse, 67–71, 231
 duties in ambulatory care, 99
 duties in emergency care, 71
 in reception center, 122, 128
Tufts University Medical Center, 47

United Kingdom, 33, 113, 167, 179, 212–213, 237
 National Health Service, 212–213, 247–248
Unecessary disability, 172, 187, 195, 197, 240
 defined, 162
Unnecessary disease, 172, 185–187, 195–198, 240
 defined, 162
Unnecessary untimely death, 172, 187, 195, 197–198, 240
 defined, 162

Veterans' Administration, 16, 219
 hospitals, 38, 40
Visiting nurse, *see* Public health nurse

Waste of professional time, 22–24, 55–58, 89, 94, 95, 109
Watts Program, Los Angeles, 88
Weed, L. L., 28
Welch, C. E., 165n